No More Diets... Ever!

The breakthrough plan that will change your life

By Carey Rossi

American Media, Inc.

NO MORE DIETS ... EVER
The breakthrough plan that will change your life

Copyright © 2004 AMI Books, Inc.
Cover design: Carlos Plaza
Interior design: Debbie Browning

ISBN: 1-932270-44-2

First printing: September 2004
Printed in the United States of America

10 9 8 7 6 5 4 3 2 1

Table of Contents

The Problem With Diets

*T*he word diet doesn't scream fun. It connotes a martinet that is all about restriction and deprivation. Think the grapefruit diet, the cabbage soup diet and the no-white food diet. Diets have become a status symbol made important by America's royalty: celebrities. Viewers of the long-running TV series *Friends* saw Rachel's physique transform from voluptuous and curvaceous to lean and toned as actress Jennifer Aniston, who played her, followed the Zone diet. Actress Renee Zellweger gained 30 pounds to play Bridget Jones and lost the weight for her next role in

Chicago by losing so much that critics called her too thin. These lives and their diets are fodder for conversations, headlines for supermarket tabloids and magazine cover blurbs. Diets have become woven into our social situations — a topic that is cool and hip.

When we see friends who have lost a lot of weight, the first thing we ask (after giving the obligatory "you look great" compliment) is "how did you do it?" I spent time at a Christmas party listening to a woman talk about how she didn't eat anything white and that she only consumed protein before noon. I also witnessed her turning up her nose at all the homemade foods that the hostess had prepared. It was difficult not to think that she was a little obsessed (and being a little bit rude). The host and hostess were followers of the Atkins diet.

Once we have been on them and have had success, we become disciples, preaching the teachings of Chopra, Atkins, Sears, Weil or any other of the new-age books of our nutritional spirituality to anyone who will listen. We forget that these diets have restricted our eating and changed our lives sometimes in good and other times in bad ways.

And here is the problem with diets. For those of us who have tried these diets and, for one reason or another, have not been able to follow their brand of nutritional logic, we should not feel as if we have failed. Instead, we should realize that the diets have failed us. There are more important things that deserve our attention. And here is where this book comes in — to get you away from the dieting cycle that can wreak havoc on your health. Researchers at the University of California at Berkeley found that women who began dieting during puberty were not only heavier than their pubescent non-dieting counterparts but they were also twice as likely to have dieted more than 20 times than those who started dieting later in life. They also found that women who had two to five moderate weight-loss episodes — losing 10 or more pounds each time — had weaker immune systems than nondieters. And the more times the women had lost the 10 or more pounds, the weaker their immune systems were.

Ultimately, your diet and exercise needs will change as you get older and your body's chemistry changes. In the course of this book you will learn how to pinpoint these changes so you can adjust accordingly.

This book is written on the premise that no matter what, you probably are not going to follow a diet with its prescribed foods and restrictions. Instead, this book is to teach you healthy eating behavior — helping you decide what types of foods are best for you and teaching you food choices that will lead you to a healthy future.

Like most people, I have tried to follow diets. I might have lasted for a week. However, I have found success by eating when I am hungry, controlling my portion sizes, living an active lifestyle and recognizing my trigger foods. I also recognize the reasons why I eat and what my relationship with food is. My weight may fluctuate now and then but when it does, I troubleshoot. As a result, my life isn't dictated by food and I have a healthy outlook on my weight and eating. This book is meant for you to be able to have the same relationship with food and yourself.

Each chapter is broken into nutritional situations or food that most of us encounter each day. Instead of quitting everything cold turkey and trying to do everything at once, you will face a chapter each week. During that week, you will set a goal to adopt a behavior that correlates to that week's topic. I will give you a sample goal but this works much better if you take the information I provide for you and set your own goal since we all have different lifestyles. Try not to move on to the next chapter until you have completed your goal for the current week since I have organized this book so that each behavior builds on another. Once you have mastered these simple eating habits, you should never feel the need to jump on the fad-diet fanfare again because diets are no way to experience life — under restrictions and rules that may not apply to you. Here you will learn to write your own rules.

Writing Your Own Rules

Setting goals are an important aspect of this book. But trying to achieve spectacular results at the outset won't get you anywhere. At the end of each chapter, you will write down a goal pertaining to what you have just learned. There are some things you should know before setting up the hurdles you want to clear for the week. Follow these guidelines suggested by sports psychologist Blair Whitmarsh, Ph.D., to ensure your success each week:

Set difficult but realistic goals. Research shows that the more difficult the goal the better the performance. However, this is only possible if the goal is realistic. Trying to achieve an unrealistic goal will only result in frustration — or worse, failure.

Set specific, measurable goals. The more specific and measurable your goals are, the easier they will be to facilitate. This should be easy based on the way this book is set up. In general, you must be able to review your goals and know whether you reached them. This includes identifying target dates for completion.

Be positive. An optimistic outlook will get you far in life and writing down your goals is no different. You will find that they are more effective and motivating when they are positive. An example of this is: "I will eat three pieces of fruit each day this week." Whitmarsh says: "Identify behaviors that you want to display as opposed to behaviors you do not want displayed. This will help you focus on what you need to do to achieve success rather than focusing on what to do to avoid failure."

Make a game plan. Identify the ways that you will attain your goal. By outlining steps on how you can achieve your desired outcome, you do all of the difficult thinking before you must do the action. In each chapter, I have outlined action steps to help you reach your week's goal and adopt that week's behavior. Once you have mastered one behavior, keep it throughout the weeks and beyond.

Why Do We Eat?

It is necessary from the time we are born. To nourish our bodies so we can grow, we eat. As babies we cry out when we are hungry and as toddlers we cry to our parents to feed us. There were times when we were told when to eat and how much. Do you remember being told to clean your plate? My parents had that rule. Since I used to eat in my room in front of the TV (I hated watching the same shows as my parents) I remember flushing brussels sprouts down the toilet to "clean my plate." I hated brussels sprouts as a child. Today, I love them.

As our tastes change, so do our reasons for eating. Just to survive or because we are hungry aren't the only reasons anymore. Our relationships with food become the overriding mechanisms of dictating when, where, what and even how much we feed ourselves. We eat because it is social, we eat because it calms our emotions and, lastly, we eat because we are hungry. Understanding the reasons why we feed ourselves and make the food choices that we do helps us come to peace with food and, eventually, never have the need to diet again. Below you will read scenarios about why others eat. You may identify with their comments and you may not. But they represent the biological, social or behavioral reasons why we eat.

The Biology of Eating

I eat for energy to make it through the day. Also, I believe it keeps your metabolism moving to burn fat. I'm old and I've been at this "weight" thing for a long time. And there is always the fact that I like to chew.

— Nikki

I am trying to watch my eating habits and I usually eat when my stomach tells me to. I don't eat much in the morning but I eat a little at lunch and watch the amount I eat at night. I do find, though, that I [do best if I] eat a small snack at night, which keeps my stomach silent. I'm doing this with exercise now to lose weight and so far have only lost about 10 pounds — not much but it's a start.

    – Pat

Sometimes because I get dizzy and/or cranky if I don't eat. Sometimes because I'm cooking and it just looks good. So I either "taste" to make sure it comes out right or actually eat even when I'm not necessarily hungry because it looks good.

    – Devin

Eating provides energy to our bodies. Simply, we take in food, the body metabolizes it into a useful substance that it can use to fuel the basic functions that allow us to live — breathing, organ functioning and flowing blood through our bodies. This is the simplest reason why we eat. It is biological.

How Food Fuels Your Body

How much energy our bodies use is determined by three factors: basal metabolic rate, physical activity and thermogenesis (heat generation).

A majority of our energy expenditure is through our basal metabolic rate, which aids the normal bodily functions that are described above. Although it is relatively consistent, it is also determined by a number of factors. How large or small our body size is the most important of these factors. The larger a person is, the higher his or her basal metabolic rate because he or she has more tissue to keep alive and generating. Another factor is body composition. Even when you are not in motion, muscle tissue requires more energy than fat. Therefore, the basal metabolic rate of a lean person is higher than that of a person that carries more fat on his or her body. As we grow older, our basal metabolic rate tends to slow for no apparent reason and we begin to notice that we are gaining more weight, even though our eating habits may not have changed.

Next is the energy we need to sustain physical activity. The factor surrounding the amount of energy needed is directly related to the intensity and the duration of the activity.

Lastly, the small component of energy output is thermogenesis, or the heat produced in response to being in a cold environment and for the digestion and absorption of a meal.

When our energy input is less than our output, weight loss is achieved. When we are consuming more than our body is using, weight gain happens. For the most part, body weight remains constant over time — meaning that our bodies have the remarkable ability to keep the balance of energy in check. Hunger drives this function. It is your body's way of signaling that it needs more energy to continue. Think about days when you are more active or when you start a new exercise program. Usually you notice that you're hungrier on those days. It is your body calling for more energy; just as you did when you were a child calling to your mother. The problem comes when these hunger signals, which will be discussed later, get clouded by such things as emotions, social events or behaviors that we have learned to associate with food.

Determining Your Body's Setpoint

Have you ever made the commitment to lose weight and stick to a strict diet only to watch helplessly as you find that at a certain weight your efforts plateau and, in the worst-case scenario, the pounds drift back?

"That must be how your body's most comfortable," your family and friends probably said in an effort to sympathize. Sounds like a well-worn excuse, but your body may have indeed gone into "famine" mode and then increased your hunger so that your body rebounds to your original weight.

Your personal level of body fat is kept within a tight range, just like your body temperature and blood sugar. Any attempt to go much above or below your body's set weight range (fatter or thinner) may be met with resistance, especially if it is rushed. Obviously, this can be a real problem if your setpoint is stuck at "a bit around the hips and thighs" or "a bit of a spare tire." In this case, you will struggle to lose weight and this fat loss will be temporary unless you combine vigilance, discipline and the setpoint-adjusting strategies outlined in this book.

Your Weight-Regulating System

To determine where your weight currently falls in relation to your setpoint, ask yourself the following questions:

● *At what weight does my body seem most "comfortable" (this isn't necessarily your ideal weight)?*

● *Is there a particular weight my body tends to climb back to after weight loss? If so, what is it?*

● *What is the heaviest I have ever weighed?*

Your answers should give you a good indication of what your metabolic setpoint weight is. You may even find that one or more setpoint weights are possible. If not, your setpoint may be more flexible than average, as setpoint stickiness — the strength of your body's resistance to dieting or overeating — varies.

Once you've guessed what your setpoint weight is, find out how many pounds above or below that weight you are right now by subtracting your setpoint weight from your current weight. Even though the natural tendency is for people to lose weight and gain it back, there are ways to lower your setpoint. The key is to get down to your desired weight and then do what you need to do to keep the weight off. If your goal is below the numbers that the above questions revealed, realize that if your final goal is more than 10 pounds below that weight, it will take as much dedication and diligence to maintain that weight as it did to lose it.

When you lose weight too quickly, your body fights back by lowering metabolism to defend its setpoint level. The effect can be dramatic: An overweight person who has lost a lot of mass through dieting may actually burn fewer calories than someone of normal weight, as one study showed. A group of non-obese men and women who weighed an average of 138 pounds needed about 2,280 calories per day to maintain their weight. A group of obese men and women weighing an average of 335 pounds needed 3,651 calories per day, but when they dieted down to 220 pounds, they needed only 2,171 calories a day to maintain this new weight — about 100 calories fewer than the lead subjects. The metabolisms of the formerly obese subjects were depressed by dieting below the level of a 138-pound non-obese individual.

While some of the decrease of metabolism was due to muscle loss, which could have been prevented if the subjects had lifted weights and eaten a significant amount of protein per pound of body weight each day, sluggishness was found to be the cause. You see, your body will drastically lower its rate of calorie burn — essentially go into famine mode — if you lose weight too quickly. That's why a gradual approach to fat loss is recommended and preferable.

Normal Calorie

The chart below lists the calorie counts the weight and the body fat listed.

Body Weight	Percentage Body Fat		
	10%	15%	20%
100	1879	1806	1732
110	2012	1931	1850
120	2144	2056	1968
130	2277	2181	2085
140	2409	2306	2203
150	2542	2431	2321
160	2674	2556	2439
170	2806	2681	2556
180	2939	2806	2674
190	3071	2931	2792
200	3204	3057	2909

Maintenance Levels

needed by a 20-year-old woman to maintain

25%	30%	35%	40%
1659	1585	1511	1438
1769	1688	1607	1526
1879	1791	1703	1614
1990	1894	1798	1703
2100	1997	1894	1791
2210	2100	1990	1879
2321	2203	2085	1968
2431	2306	2181	2056
2542	2409	2277	2144
2652	2512	2372	2233
2762	2615	2468	2321

Rowley, B. Winning the Weight-Loss Game.
Muscle & Fitness Hers, December 2002/January 2003.
Reprinted with permission

Interestingly, genetic differences in setpoint stickiness — the strength of your body's resistance to dieting or overeating — explains why some people are at risk for getting fat while others aren't. When test subjects were fed 1,000 calories per day above what they needed to stay at their current weight for 12 weeks, they gained different amounts of weight, from 9 to 29 pounds. Pairs of twins with sticky setpoints burned most of the extra calories by fidgeting, up to an incredible 700 calories per day, and gained less weight over the 12 weeks. This research suggests that genetics play an important role in obesity.

Discoveries of complex and interwoven hormone pathways regulating appetite, fat metabolism, fat production and fat breakdown also suggest a more biological basis for the setpoint. Neuropeptide Y, leptin, melanin-concentrating hormone, cholecystokinin, norepinephrine and serotonin are hormones that regulate body fatness. Each one also has a receptor to which it binds, making things even more complicated.

One primary factor in predicting who will get fat and who won't is respiratory quotient — a measure of how much of the energy a body burns in a day comes from carbohydrates versus fats. People with high respiratory quotients burn proportionately more carbs and conserve fats, while those with low respiratory quotients burn more fats and fewer carbs. According to Robert Pool, author of *Fat: Fighting the Obesity Epidemic*, scientists report that people with the highest respiratory quotients are more than twice as likely to gain 11 or more pounds over the next two to four years as people with the lowest respiratory quotients. Women, who tend to burn less and store more fat than men, may fall in the former category more often.

The Emotional Side of Eating

I eat if I want to reward myself — e.g., I had a bad day so I pick up a pint of Ben & Jerry's ice cream on the way home because, damn it, I deserve it!
– Natasha

Sometimes I eat because I'm in my "eating place," i.e. the couch, and it's nighttime. It just feels like I need to eat

*when I'm there, kind of a ritual like
brushing my teeth at the end of the day.*
    – Michelle

At some point in our lives, we associated food with comfort — a safe activity that provides solace from life's pressures. In a society where high-fat food is thought to be off-limits, we have associated the pleasant foods of our childhood as rewards.

Emotional distress is frequently accompanied by overeating. Food can be used for self-medicating purposes and, when consumed in excess over time, can prompt the same brain activity that results from drug abuse. For instance, binge eating is often triggered by the ingestion of small amounts of food. This parallels the priming effect of drugs in addicts whereby even a small dose elicits a strong craving and compulsion for further use. A key vulnerability in this behavior is a "sensitivity to reward," which is a psychobiological trait that involves the dopamine pathways that are in the mesolimbic area of the brain. This is the area that controls memory and emotion. Researchers at York University in Toronto, Ontario, Canada, found that those who have a high sensitivity to reward tend to increase their eating when feeling depressed more than their less sensitive counterparts. What is interesting is they found that these same subjects did not overeat when faced with other negative emotions, like anger, frustration or anxiety. They also found that emotional eating had a significant relationship with body mass index, demonstrating that the obese tend to overeat more than the overweight subjects who, in turn, tend to overeat more than their normal weight counterparts.

Eating has become an easy, cheap reward that gives instant gratification. If you find yourself eating large amounts of food to make yourself feel better then it is time to look at why you are eating. Let me share a little story with you.

When I was 22, I got my first job in a surf town in the central California coast. I knew no one and was working about 12 hours a day managing a restaurant. I have always loved ice cream and on a hot summer day I decided to pick up a pint of Ben & Jerry's while grocery shopping. No big deal really. That night, I decide to indulge in my treat by eating it straight from the carton. After eating for a little while I realized that I had downed half the pint — more than I intended. I put it back into the freezer. Within five minutes I had retrieved it and was eating more. This time I felt driven to reach the bottom. Of course, I did and I was so nauseous. This began a year of this ice cream bingeing behavior every day. I lived between two convenience stores that carried Ben & Jerry's, so I would alternate which one I would walk to each day. The catch was that I had to walk to go get my pint because then, at least, I was exercising.

When I started gaining weight, I would go to the gym and walk on the treadmill for two hours because I had to purge the extra 1,000 or so calories I was eating per day (sometimes 2,000 if I had eaten two pints!). Too young to realize I was depressed about my living, work and now my weight situation, I really didn't realize why I continued to secretly eat my weight in Ben & Jerry's ice cream. Finally, I was transferred to Orange County. I decided then never to have ice cream again. I continued to work out and I watched what I ate. I even realized that pasta made me crave ice cream, so I cut that out. After a year, I lost my B&J weight. Now, I still crave ice cream when I am depressed. But the difference is I can see it. Sometimes you can't see it or identify it until you have separated yourself. In the chapter about food journaling, keep your eyes open for the emotional behaviors that spur your food choices.

The Social Aspect of Eating

I eat to be social, i.e., at lunch with colleagues, at dinner with friends/colleagues, sitting down for a snack to take a break from shopping with friends or to accompany certain activities (e.g., popcorn or candy at a movie, scone or muffin while reading the paper in Starbucks).

— Natasha

I realized my girlfriend and I often eat just for the social aspects — the reason to go out. I noticed that I like to go out not so much for the food itself, but because it gives us a reason to do something.

Now, I know technically it should be possible to eat out and eat healthy, but honestly, most restaurants don't make it easy. Unless you really like salad, you're in trouble (and it's hard to avoid the temptations when you're in a place with a menu full of goodies).

Social eating is a real dilemma — it's hard to simply say, "I'm going to stop eating out." For us, for instance, if we do that, what's the replacement? We lose our destination. I think a lot of people are in the same boat; there isn't a ton of things an adult couple can do socially that are fun and don't revolve around food.

— Michael

There is a line in the movie *When Harry Met Sally* when Sally's friend quotes a magazine article that she had read — something to the effect that restaurants are to the '80s what theater used to be in the '70s. Restaurants have become the destination of evenings out with loved ones and friends. If you live in cities that have a "culinary" scene, you may find that restaurants come and go with the times. Journalist Jeffrey Kluger described it best in his *Time* magazine article about why we eat: "The act of pulling up and tucking in, of passing around and helping oneself is one of the most primal of shared activities. We eat together when we celebrate and we eat together when we grieve; we eat together when a loved one is preparing to leave, and we eat together when the loved one returns. We solve our problems over the family dinner table, conduct our business over the executive lunch table and entertain guests over cake and cookies at the coffee table."

Food has become the centerpiece of our social existence. It even helps complete the experiences. I live in Los Angeles and it is almost a ritual to have a "Dodger dog" when you go see a game in Chavez ravine. Other friends that I spoke to about why we eat say that it is sometimes just part of a full experience. For instance, they must have popcorn or it's not really a movie, or they must have cake at a birthday party. There are many holidays that involve food; for instance, Thanksgiving. How many times do you walk away from a Thanksgiving table feeling as stuffed as the turkey that you just ate? In our cultural melting pot, there are many religions that dictate what to eat and how to eat. For example, kosher Jews do not eat shellfish or pork and do not mix dairy and meat.

Numerous studies have demonstrated that people eat larger amounts of food when they eat in the presence of others than when they eat alone. This social facilitation of eating occurs no matter the time of day, whether or not alcohol is consumed, which particular meal is being eaten, whether the eating takes place on the weekend or the weekday or whether the eating occurs at a restaurant or elsewhere.

However, the amount of food consumed in front of others doesn't always mean that more food will be consumed. The presence of others can inhibit eating in a variety of circumstances: when their company is not eating but merely watching; when the importance of acceptance of the others is high (i.e., you are aware of the type of impression you want to make and, therefore, you are acting accordingly) and when the others are not eating a lot. This is a form of modeling or conformity that dictates our eating patterns. As such, research studies have consistently found the participants eat very little when their eating partners do so. However, when their eating partners eat large amounts of food, the naïve participants in the study also eat large quantities of the food. When they are left to their own devices without others to set the amount of food, they eat intermediate amounts of food. This may be because in certain situations, we may look to others to dictate th correct or appropriate amount to consume. The influences of social eating on the amount of food we consume were studied by researchers at the University of Toronto at Mississauga. Participants in the study ate more when they were led to believe that the person at the table before them ate more. They ate less when they were led to believe that the prior person ate less or when they were not provided any information about the eating habits of the prior person.

It may be that the food choices we make are also influenced by socialization. As discussed earlier, individuals' food choices reflect their cultural backgrounds and thus demonstrate the family resemblance in food preferences. It is assumed that one of the factors in food choices is the imitation of our parent's nutritional habits and choices as we are growing up.

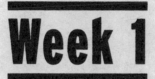

Week 1

Getting Comfortable in Your Skin

When I worked in magazines, graphic artists would use a computer program called Photoshop to trim waists and thighs or even create a six-pack from a pouchy stomach. During that time, I felt the pressure to be thin for public appearances. I felt that as an editor of a women's fitness magazine I had to represent the images that were represented on my pages even though I am 5-foot-nothing and about 120 pounds.

Self-esteem is a positive or negative orientation toward oneself: an overall evaluation of one's worth or value.
– Murat Sahin Alagoz, M.D., Ayse Devrim Basterzi, M.D., Ahmet Cagri Uysal, M.D., et al. in *Aesthetic Plastic Surgery* 2003

It wasn't that I disliked myself — I was just aware of my place in that publishing world. Otherwise, I had and still do have a good outlook on my life, my appearance and me. In the big picture of self-esteem, body image is only a part of it — how you internally view your outer being. In some cases it may help, but if you think little of who you are and the person that you are becoming, you should be reading a self-help book. You can't lose weight unless you are comfortable with the situations around you. The fact is that you may have gained the weight because of them.

Body image is dynamic, changing with time and is affected by internal as well as external factors.
– Alagoz et al.

As I write this, I remember all of the healthy eating behaviors that I have learned over the course of my life — either from my own parents, the fitness magazines I read as a teen or the fitness magazines I edited as an adult. My point is that circumstances can influence our thoughts — whether it's politics, music or even about how we feel about ourselves. Our opinions ebb and flow depending on the moon cycle, hormones, whether the sun is shining or just how great — or not — we are feeling.

When making the decision to commit to lose weight and eat healthier, knowing what your frame of mind is at the time is paramount. After all, if it is a fleeting thought, your efforts will be fleeting, as well. You may even fail. And that will just begin another cycle of dieting that you are trying to avoid. It may have even been the reason why you decided to pick up this book in the first place.

Much of how we view our bodies comes from how other people — family, friends, significant others and spouses — relate to us and our bodies starting in our earliest years. According to ongoing studies, your body image could be the result of your parents' behavior and their comments regarding weight-loss issues, such as diet and exercise. In fact, your mom might have unwittingly been the first to teach you the stereotypes of thinness and beauty that plague our society.

Parenting isn't an exact science so it may not surprise you to know that mothers and fathers make a direct contribution to the body image bank. Preoccupied with their weight and sometimes that of their spouses, parents might be subconsciously passing these behaviors on to their children. You may have adopted some of these bad-body thoughts as young as age 8. This includes the negative self-talk that you may hear when you are looking in the mirror.

Researchers at Kenyon College in Gambier, Ohio, studied fourth- and fifth-graders and their parents. They found that daughters whose parents expressed weight concerns were dissatisfied with their bodies. Also, they discovered that a mother's comments about her daughter's weight were significantly related to the latter's attempts to lose weight. Father's comments were not seen as a significant influence alone but when combined with the mother's comments, it tended to exacerbate the problem. This same study also found that girls received more feedback than boys and that was associated with poor body image.

As we move into adulthood such body-conscious criticism doesn't stop having an effect on us. The Universities of Central Florida and South Florida asked female and male undergraduates to recall any feedback from either parent about their appearance as it related to their body images. Findings indicated that mothers were more likely than fathers to comment on appearance, affecting the students' body images into adulthood.

As we get older, we develop relationships with men and women who shape our world. They help alleviate some of the world's pressures but they also introduce their own pressure — to look good, to be thin and maybe influence the way that you view your appearance. Boyfriends or girlfriends can impose their appearance beliefs on you. Enough coffee talk or drinks with friends where everyone is having a pity party about your beer belly can alter your outlook on yourself. These relationships are one of the least scientifically explored in terms of body image. Though not investigated, these relationships are important to us — the desire to be accepted and evaluated by others.

What effect do others have on your body image?

Ask yourself the following questions to see whether your body image is affected by the people around you.

● *Is your mother concerned with whether you weigh too much or may someday?*

● *Is your father concerned with whether you weigh too much or may someday?*

● *Is your significant other/spouse concerned with whether you weigh too much or may someday?*

● *How important is it to your mother that you are thin?*

● *How important is it to your father that you are attractive?*

● *How important is it to your significant other/spouse that you are attractive?*

● *Does your mother diet often?*

● *Does your mother pay a lot of attention to her appearance?*

● *How many friends want to be thinner or make a significant change to their appearance?*

● *Do you and your friends complain that you're fat?*

Adapted from M.P. Levine, L. Smolak, and H. Hayden. "Parent Involvement Scale, Mother Influence Scale and Peer Dieting Scale." *Exacting Beauty: Theory, Assessment, and Treatment of Body Image Disturbance.* Eds. J. Kevin Thompson, Leslie J. Heinberg, Madeline Altabe, and Stacy Tantleff-Dunn. American Psychological Association: Washington, D.C., 1999, p. 202-204.

Our environment can also have a lot to do with how we evaluate ourselves. In my example about how I used to diet before my public appearances, I did it mostly because I would be around models and fitness competitors who were as tall as I am but smaller than me. I always felt like a giant next to them. Since I am usually smaller than everyone around me, this made me extremely uncomfortable. Being in an environment where everyone's body fat percentage was in the teens (not healthy for women and I do not recommend it) made me feel critical of my body. Such feelings of being uncomfortable in our environment can have a powerful influence on our psyche. If you live in a place where most of the people are thin and active, you may feel the pressure to conform.

Society can provide the pressures, except the norms tend to be fickle and ever-changing. For instance, the ideals of beauty for women have ranged from thin and skinny that is unattainable for many and only accomplished by starvation, to lean, muscular and large breasts that is unattainable without restrictive dieting, excessive exercise and breast augmentation. Currently, the celebrity bodies of Jennifer Lopez and Beyonce Knowles have changed the acceptability of bodies that have a bit more in the backside. But according to an article in *W* magazine called "The S-Curve," the new physique of 2004 is the body that has an ample bosom, a slim taut waist, a bubble butt and tight, toned legs. Let's talk about impossible ideal. While there is no concrete evidence to measure the amount of influence that the media have over how we measure our self-worth, one has to wonder whether Beyonce's bootylicious behind has made it acceptable for us to feel better about the average American's widening backside. Numerous studies have been performed that measure women's self-esteem after reading fashion magazines and, in most cases, the undergraduates that are the participants feel worse about their bodies immediately afterward. To measure for yourself the effect that society has on your self-esteem, take the following questionnaire now. Then retake it after reading a fashion or fitness magazine, watching your favorite television show, or after seeing a movie starring your favorite actor or actress. Compare your answers and see if there is a difference.

What Is My Self-Esteem?

Answer the following questions to determine your self-esteem.

1. *Do you like what you look like in pictures?*

2. *Do you think others consider you good-looking?*

3. *Are you proud of your body?*

4. *Do you think you can get a job because of your appearance?*

5. *When you look in a mirror, do you like the person you see?*

6. *Are there lots of things that you would change about your appearance?*

7. *Are you satisfied with your weight?*

8. *Do you wish you were more handsome or pretty?*

9. *Are you comfortable with your body shape?*

10. *Do you wish you looked like someone else?*

11. *Do your peers like what you look like?*

12. *Are you happy with your appearance?*

13. *Do you ever feel ashamed about how you look? If so, how often?*

14. *Does stepping on the scale depress you?*

15. *Does your body's shape depress you?*

16. *Are you able to garner attention from your preferred sex?*

17. *Do you worry about the way you look?*

18. *Do you like your body's shape?*

19. *Do you feel that you look the best that you can?*

20. *Do you feel comfortable with your body when you are naked?*

Adapted from B.K. Mendelson. "Body-Esteem Scale

for Adolescents and Adults." *Exacting Beauty: Theory, Assessment, and Treatment of Body Image Disturbance.* Eds. J. Kevin Thompson, Leslie J. Heinberg, Madeline Altabe, and Stacy Tantleff-Dunn. American Psychological Association: Washington, DC., 1999, p. 80.

Look at your answers to the questions. Which ones did you answer yes? Which ones did you answer no? If you want to look like someone else, or your looks depress you or make you ashamed or worried, then it is time to work on your self-esteem.

Before losing the extra weight, you need to thwart your own body-image devils. Use the information that you have gathered from the previous sets of questions to change your image of yourself. The most effective approach to do so is a cognitive-behavior strategy. This intervention explores the origin of body-image distur-bances and attempts to eliminate these feelings through a multistep program. *The Body Image Workbook: An 8-Step Program* (MJF Books, 1997) by Thomas F. Cash, Ph.D., is considered a highly effective example of this methodology. In his book, Cash helps the reader explore the origins of body-image disturbances and how to overcome those influences by leading you through the following steps: exploring your own body image; setting goals to change it; identifying your perceptions about your body and its image; correcting your inner voice; facing your fears and destroying self-defecting rituals; rewarding your body with affirming and enhancing activities, and learning to be comfortable with your body.

Week 1 Getting Comfortable Goals:

This week, take the quizzes in this chapter and really examine why you answered the way that you did. Create action plans on ways to thwart negative self-talk.

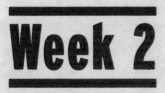

Week 2

Starting
Your Journal

Now that you understand all of the mechanisms that affect the way we eat, it's time to examine how, what and why you specifically eat. Since we are not all the same and because each person faces his or her own stresses and social obligations, why, when, what and how we eat is very different. To establish your own healthy eating behavior, it is important to understand your eating habits and the situations surrounding them. To do this, keep a food journal.

There are always so many factors surrounding eating. If you really want to become healthier or even lose some weight, it is important to recognize these factors and how they influence what goes into your mouth. One of the most successful techniques for weight loss is self-monitoring. This is when a person tracks and analyzes his or her behaviors, usually in a journal.

Because this book is about changing your eating behaviors so that you no longer need to think about or rely on diets, you will begin keeping a food journal now.

Start by taking 12 days out of the next month to keep a food journal. To do this, pick three days each week. Mix up the days so that sometimes they are consecutive and other times they are not, that some days are weekdays and others are weekends and that some days are stressful and others are carefree. By documenting so many days in a month, hopefully you will be keeping track of a variety of situations that accurately portray your life and how you fuel yourself during it. Before you think "What a pain!" don't see it as an exercise in self-deprecation or a measurement of your willpower. Food journaling is a research-backed method of monitoring your food intake. You can make your journal as intricate or as personal as you want. The following are three steps to get you started.

Step One: Choose Your Vice

Personalizing your food diary enhances your chances of success. Whether it's a spiral-bound notebook, an electronic personal assistant, a Web site or a computer program, or simply photocopies of the pages at the end of this chapter, you need to use whatever will work for you. Below you will find the pros and cons of each food journaling method. And at this chapter's end, you will find sample journal pages you can use to achieve this week's goals.

Type of food journal: Paper journals

Advantages: Easy to use and small enough to fit in a purse, wallet or pocket. You could use a little spiral notebook, a nice journal or even a pocket calendar.

● It can be as detailed or as abbreviated as you want.

● It is easy to flip through for comparison and identifying patterns.

Disadvantages: You'll need to consult a nutrition book to figure out calories and nutrients of foods.

● Daily totals aren't calculated automatically.

Type of food journal: PDA programs
Advantages: Small enough to take with you almost anywhere.

● Calculates daily calorie and nutrient totals automatically.

Disadvantages: Can take a long time to program new foods.

● Downloading the software can be frustrating if you are not apt to it.

● Food database can be small.

Type of food journal: Internet programs
Advantages: Large database of foods to choose from.

● Many free programs are available.

● Some programs can also create diet programs for you.

Disadvantages: You can't carry it with you.

● You may have to keep records on paper and then enter it to the site and, therefore, you may not enter in everything.

Step Two: Details, Details, Details

Researchers at Brown University's Weight Control and Diabetes Research Center in Providence, Rhode Island, put two groups of dieting women on either a detailed or more simplified food diary protocol. Those who kept the more detailed diary lost about twice as much weight as those who kept the abbreviated diaries. This could signify that the more detailed your food journal, the more success you will have in making the changes you are hoping to.

Like everything in this book, take everything in moderation. This includes self-monitoring. Start by just recording the food you are eating and the time you are eating (for example: 7 a.m.: 1 packet of maple and brown sugar oatmeal, 1 cup orange juice). Then, add where you are eating it. The next week, keep track of how you are eating: Are you eating quickly or are you savoring every bite? Lastly, start recording why you are eating: Are you hungry? Bored? Tired? Satisfying a craving?

After writing down approximations of the foods you're eating, you may want to start writing down the details. Get specific with food measurement and preparation. Instead of writing "chicken," you would write "10-ounces grilled chicken." The Internet can be a great source to help with calorie counts and restaurant Web sites often list their nutritional information.

Step Three: Tell the Truth

We lie to hide — hide from getting in trouble, hide from being blamed and hide to look good. When you lie to your food journal, you are lying to yourself — especially when you don't record the binges on Ben & Jerry's ice cream or the all-day chocolate fest you indulged in. When you don't record these occurrences and the reasons behind them, you will forget about them. Most importantly, you won't learn from them. Journaling isn't about "behaving"; it is about monitoring your actions — the good and the bad. A food diary is only as effective as you are honest with it.

Sometimes the whole process does get frustrating. For instance, you're recording your food and you aren't losing weight even though your diary says you should. The problem might be that you aren't logging in everything. You know, the handful of M&Ms from your co-worker's candy jar or that regular soda you had while you were shopping. All of these things add up.

On the other end of the spectrum, if you aren't truthful about any bingeing or snacking activity you may have, then you might be hiding a much larger problem that could be a result of your environment. Remember this program isn't a diet. It's a way to live healthfully. You can't be healthy if you don't see or understand your actions. The simple act of writing all of this down will make you more aware of your actions and your behaviors.

Example Week 2 Goal: I will record all meals and snacks on Tuesday, Thursday and Saturday of this week.

Your Week 2 Goal:

_____

_____

_____

_____

_____

_____

Food Journal Game Plan:

● Use sample diary No. 1 — either photocopy or recreate it — and carry it with you. Record all meals immediately afterward.

● Do you use a notebook or a pad for work? Use the last few pages to record the food you are eating.

● Preset single-serving packaging makes food journaling a snap. Added benefit is that you will learn proper portions (but that will also come later).

● Remember this isn't about being a good eater or a bad eater; it's about learning how, what, where, why and when you eat. Having this understanding will pave the way for healthy behaviors down the road.

Sample Nutrition

Copy these pages to keep track of what you eat
will help you be more mindful of what you put
of calories you consume each day, use a calorie-

	Breakfast	Lunch	Dinner
Monday			
Tuesday			
Wednesday			
Thursday			
Friday			
Saturday			
Sunday			

Diary No. 1

each week. Writing down everything you eat
in your mouth. To help calculate the number
counting book available at your local bookstore.

Snack 1	Snack 2	Water Intake	Total Daily Calories

Sample Nutrition

Copy these pages to keep track of what you eat
will help you be more mindful of what you put
of calories you consume each day, use a calorie-

	Breakfast	Lunch	Dinner
Monday			
Tuesday			
Wednesday			
Thursday			
Friday			
Saturday			
Sunday			

Diary No. 1

each week. Writing down everything you eat in your mouth. To help calculate the number counting book available at your local bookstore.

Snack 1	Snack 2	Water Intake	Total Daily Calories

Sample Nutrition

Copy these pages to keep track of what you eat
will help you be more mindful of what you put
of calories you consume each day, use a calorie-

	Breakfast	Lunch	Dinner
Monday			
Tuesday			
Wednesday			
Thursday			
Friday			
Saturday			
Sunday			

Diary No. 1

each week. Writing down everything you eat
in your mouth. To help calculate the number
counting book available at your local bookstore.

Snack 1	Snack 2	Water Intake	Total Daily Calories

Sample Nutrition

Copy these pages to keep track of what you eat
will help you be more mindful of what you put
eat, what you eat, how much you eat, where
mood is, you can identify patterns to your eating
you consume each day, use a calorie-counting

Today's date is:

Meal/Snack	Time	Description

Diary No. 2

each day. Writing down everything you eat
in your mouth. By writing down when you
you eat, how hungry you are and what your
habits. To help calculate the number of calories
book available at your local bookstore.

Amount	Location	Hunger Level	Mood

Sample Nutrition

Copy these pages to keep track of what you eat
will help you be more mindful of what you put
eat, what you eat, how much you eat, where
mood is, you can identify patterns to your eating
you consume each day, use a calorie-counting

Today's date is:

Meal/Snack	Time	Description

Diary No. 2

each day. Writing down everything you eat
in your mouth. By writing down when you
you eat, how hungry you are and what your
habits. To help calculate the number of calories
book available at your local bookstore.

Amount	Location	Hunger Level	Mood

Sample Nutrition

Copy these pages to keep track of what you eat
will help you be more mindful of what you put
eat, what you eat, how much you eat, where
mood is, you can identify patterns to your eating
you consume each day, use a calorie-counting

Today's date is:

Meal/Snack	Time	Description

Diary No. 2

each day. Writing down everything you eat
in your mouth. By writing down when you
you eat, how hungry you are and what your
habits. To help calculate the number of calories
book available at your local bookstore.

Amount	Location	Hunger Level	Mood

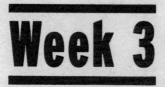

Honing In on Your Hunger

The best way to decide how much and when to eat is to listen to your body. Our body's hunger signals can dictate when it is time to eat. The problem occurs when we don't listen to those signals or we misread other things like boredom as hunger. By understanding your hunger signals, the whole calorie-counting business could be disregarded. Think about it: Simply eat according to physical hunger and fullness. Too bad it isn't that simple.

Trying to decide if our sweet cravings after a meal are physical or psychological can be difficult to decipher. How many times do we ignore these signals of hunger because food isn't available when our stomachs are growling or eat more than we should because it tastes so good? The following will tell you how to read your hunger signals.

To Eat or Not to Eat

Mechanisms that control eating behavior fall into two very broad categories: eating signals and non-eating signals. Hunger and appetite are the big eating signals; satiation and satiety are the main non-eating signals.

Eating signals. Hunger is a primarily physical sensation that drives your need to eat. You may know these signals as a grumbling stomach, difficulty concentrating or other strong physiological signs. A desire to eat or an appetite can occur with or without hunger.

Non-eating signals. When you are full from a meal and you have decided to stop eating, you are experiencing satiation. Satiety is how long you stay full.

A long list of hormones and physical mechanisms trigger hunger and satiety. But in the end, appetite is what most often determines how much we eat.

Measuring Your Appetite

Some nutrition experts believe one answer to weight management lies in letting internal hunger and satiety cues rather than external appetite cues determine what to eat. A hunger scale is often recommended to help "reconnect" with your body's natural cues.

Think about how your body talks to you. Start paying attention to how your body begins to tell you that you are hungry and, eventually, lets you know that you need to eat *now*. After you fully understand these feelings, you can use a hunger scale to help your decision process of whether you should eat. You can look at these feelings as increments of 0 to 10. Zero signifies "Thanksgiving full" and 10 means "extremely hungry." Think of numbers 0 to 4 as the numbers of satiation and satiety and the numbers of 8 to 10 as the numbers of hunger. The numbers of 5 to 7 form the transition area of your hunger scale.

Create the best scale that works for you. It doesn't have to be a 10-point scale. Make the scale fit into your body's communication system. Use this scale in your food journal. It will help you decipher whether you are eating when you are hungry or not.

Filling Up?

Research shows that calories are the bottom line in achieving satiation rather than the weight of food or beverages, a food's fiber content, the speed of eating or drinking or having a protein, carbohydrate and/or fat in a meal. Researchers at Purdue University in West Lafayette, Indiana, compared the hunger ratings of subjects who had consumed a variety of foods at different times. They found that hunger ratings were the lowest after consuming food portions of 500 calories. The bottom line is that if you haven't had enough calories, your hunger will return quickly.

The makeup of your meal will also determine how long you will be satiated. Meals that have a mixture of carbohydrates, protein and fats will keep you fuller longer. The body digests carbohydrates first, then proteins and last fats. If your meal is mostly carbohydrates, you will find that you're hungry sooner than if your meal features a combination of macronutrients.

Food Form

The form of food — solid, semi-solid or liquid — may greatly influence satiety signals. In particular, liquid calories don't seem to sate us like solid food does because they do not trigger the cues. For example, if you have a regular cola with your lunch, most likely you are not going to eat less of your lunch as a result. Solid foods allow for you to adjust your consumption of calories; if not at the time that you are eating, definitely later in the day.

Foods like milkshakes, smoothies and blended coffee drinks are considered semi-solid foods and fall into a satiety gray area. If you tend to consume these things, be attentive to the amount of calories you are consuming throughout the day.

Sample Week 3 Hunger Honing Goal: I will continue journaling my food intake three days this week and add hunger ratings to my entries.

Your Hunger Honing Goal:

_____

_____

_____

_____

_____

_____

Hunger Honing Game Plan

● Create hunger scale for your individual needs.

● Allow yourself to get really full and really hungry. Pay attention to how your body responds to these two extremes.

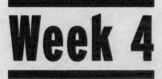

Week 4

Stop Drinking Your Calories

Your first step to losing weight without really thinking about it is to switch from caloric beverages to noncaloric ones. In a study of sugar-intake trends, researchers from the University of North Carolina at Chapel Hill found that between the years of 1977 and 1996, there was an increase in the amount of calories from sweeteners consumed — an 83-calorie per person increase. The caloric beverages that I am speaking of are sodas. These drinks provide no nutritional value and do not make you feel full. What they do is add calories to your daily caloric intake. In the previously mentioned study, 54 of those 83 calories were contributed by soda. If you are not moving to burn these calories, they can add up and turn into pounds. One might expect beverages to be helpful in lowering the amount of calories consumed throughout the day. And there seems to be no agreement to the impact of liquid calories on satiety.

Soda has become the primary thirst-quencher in the United States, but because it doesn't trigger the satiety mechanisms in our brain we continue to eat. If you were to just have one can of soda, it would be an extra 250 calories a day. In 10 days, you would weigh an extra pound. In one year, you would gain about 36 pounds. And that is only if you were to drink one can of soda per day. With the Big Gulps and the super-sodas at restaurants, who really knows the serving size of the soda you are drinking? That is why it is much easier to make the switch. This means more water but other noncaloric beverages are OK, too. Thanks to the soda companies, we have diet sodas, (Diet Coke with lime is my personal favorite) and flavored-carbonated waters that have no calories. There are also the old standbys of coffee and tea.

The New Face of Coffee

When I was growing up in Palm Springs, California, my mom would take me to The Coffee Bean and Tea Leaf. There, she would get her coffee and I would get an ice-blended mocha. For those outside of California, Nevada or Arizona, an ice-blended coffee is refreshment that borders on a milkshake. In the early 1980s, this was the ultimate treat and I usually couldn't finish it. Today, a 16-ounce ice-blended mocha is 360 calories and the grande-sized mocha frappuccino, Starbucks' equivalent, is 420 calories. It's new light version, mocha frappuccino blended coffee, is 180 calories for the grande size.

Sucking down café mochas and other creamy concoctions that have enough calories to be a meal can add the pounds quickly. If you are having a chocolate craving, eating a piece of chocolate or opting for a candy bar may be more satisfying and keep you feeling full longer. If you are looking for a coffee treat, consider ordering a flavored coffee or if that isn't available, order a small (or tall, if you are at Starbucks) nonfat latte with some sugar-free syrup. At 120 calories, it will satisfy your craving but keep your calories low.

The Fattening Side of Fruit

If your local smoothie shop knows you by name (or by drink) then you might be drinking more calories than you think. A 24-ounce smoothie from Jamba Juice or Robek's can easily consist of 400 to 500 calories and some smoothies are almost 800 calories. If you decide to gulp the jumbo sizes, you're looking at nearly 1,000 calories and possibly beyond. If you choose to juice, order the smallest size available for a snack or consider the regular size of your meal.

Taming the Soda Junkie

Quitting soda and other caloric beverages cold turkey may be difficult because they taste so good and you hate the taste of water. Use these tips to wean the Kool-Aid kid in you:

● When you are at a self-serve soda fountain, fill your cup up two-thirds of the way with diet soda and then top off the rest with your full-calorie favorite.

● Drink the diet version of your full-calorie favorite.

● Add a half- cup of fruit juice to water.

● Keep a pitcher of water with sliced oranges, limes, lemons, grapefruits, cucumbers or mint in your refrigerator. They will flavor the water for you.

● Drink beverages like Propel water from Gatorade or Crystal Light. These ultra-low-calorie drinks in large quantities still do less damage to your waistline than full-calorie soda.

● Make a pact with yourself that you will substitute a glass of water for one soda one week. The next week substitute two glasses of water for two sodas. Continue the process until you are no longer drinking soda or large amounts of any caloric drinks.

Water, Water Everywhere

How many times have we heard that we should be consuming at least eight 8-ounce glasses of water? According to the Institute of Medicine panel of U.S. and Canadian scientists, men need an average of 16 cups of water a day and women need 11 cups of water a day. But that doesn't mean you need to drink that much water. All the fluid you consume is included in that 11 or 16 cups. This means all the soda, tea, coffee, milk and even alcohol, and the moisture in foods. Tabitha Elliot, Ph.D., reported in *Muscle & Fitness* magazine that researchers also suggest that there is an extreme variability in water requirements for every individual that depends on climate, activity level and how much he or she sweats. When it comes down to it, you will do fine if you just drink when you are thirsty.

If you are trying to lose weight, the more water you drink the better. Water has no calories and makes you feel full. This means that dieters fare better the more they drink. And if you are exercising, this will increase your fluid requirements. So drink up to lose fat. An easy way to get more water is to set goals or tricks for yourself.

● Find a large glass or bottle and tell yourself that you will drink one container full of water before you can have any other type of beverage. Increase the amount of water each week.

● Use an old drinking tip: alternate beverages. Switch between water and the beverage of your choice. For example, have a cup of coffee followed by a glass of water, then maybe a diet cola followed by a glass of water.

Sample Week 4 Stop Drinking Your Calories Goals: I will drink one of these _ gallon containers of water each day and I cannot have any other liquid refreshment until it is finished.

or

I will only order diet soda or iced tea when I go out to eat.

or

I will only order regular coffee or its iced equivalent.

Your Week 4 Stop Drinking Your Calories Goals:

_____

_____

_____

_____

_____

_____

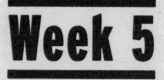

Rise and Shine! It's Time to Eat

Do you eat breakfast? If you are like most Americans, you probably don't and that's too bad. Skipping breakfast is a habit that tends to increase with age. Breakfast consumption trends reflect new behaviors rather than the changing social demographics of the United States. For instance, as watching your weight becomes more prevalent it is easier to justify skipping your morning meal no matter what the consequences.

The first meal of the day sets the tone for your eating during the rest of your day. Omitting breakfast or worse, eating an inadequate breakfast (coffee and a pastry), may contribute to nutrition inadequacies that are never replenished throughout your day.

If that isn't reason enough to set your clock 10 minutes earlier, try these:

Breakfast can improve your overall health. Research shows that individuals who consume breakfast cereal every day report better mental and physical health than those who consume breakfast less frequently. In addition, people who eat breakfast tend to have a healthier lifestyle than nonbreakfast eaters.

Breakfast can keep you alert. Sans coffee, no one food alone will perk you up for that morning meeting. Your morning meal should be high in fiber and low in fat. Ready-to-eat cereals fall into this category perfectly — a little cereal, a little milk **and** viola.

Breakfast can help you perform better. Eating first thing in the morning enhances your ability to handle mental tasks. Studies suggest that children who skip breakfast have more difficulty with cognition and working memory tasks.

Breakfast can perk up your mood. Research shows that individuals who consume a cereal breakfast each day are less depressed, less emotionally distressed and have lower levels of perceived stress than those who didn't eat breakfast each day.

Breakfast can help you manage your weight. The simple act of just eating breakfast can help keep obesity at bay. While most people skip breakfast to decrease their caloric intake for the day, it usually backfires on them — bingeing later to make up for the caloric deficiency. Research shows that individuals who consume a high-fiber cereal in the morning consume fewer calories at lunch.

Breakfast can enhance the overall quality of your diet. A healthy morning meal can set the nutrition tone of your day. Ready-to-eat cereals are traditionally thought of as breakfast fast food. Ninety-two percent of ready-to-eat cereals are fortified with essential nutrients. Therefore, they have a significant effect on your nutritional quality for the day. Researchers have found that ready-to-eat cereal consumption has been shown to result in lower daily intake of fat, saturated fat and cholesterol. (Apparently those Cheerios and oatmeal commercials are true.) Those who consume ready-to-eat cereal take in more vitamins and minerals each day than those who do not. Another plus to ready-to-eat cereal — milk. Those who consume milk with cereal tend to drink more, which means more calcium and stronger bones.

A Better Breakfast

So if you haven't figured it out, one of the first steps to take to diminish diets for good is to eat breakfast. But as stated above, coffee and a pastry or bacon and eggs just won't do. Use the checklist below to create a better breakfast:

❑ *Include calcium.* Consuming milk at breakfast usually means that you will consume enough throughout the day.

❑ *Include ready-to-eat cereal.* Quick, fast, easy cereal is the superstar of breakfast foods. Research done independently and funded by Quaker and Kellogg's has found that those who eat ready-to-eat cereal report better mental and physical health, increased consumption of essential vitamins and minerals, and lower intakes of fat and cholesterol. To get the best bang for your cereal buck, choose whole-grain cereals. These cereals are high in antioxidants (a cancer-fighting compound found in fruits and vegetables).

❑ *Make your breakfast high in fiber and carbohydrates and low in fat.* A high-fiber and carbohydrate, low-fat meal will keep you satiated longer than a high-fat, high-protein meal. This combination is the most effective in curbing your appetite for a longer period of time. On the other hand, a high-fat breakfast is most likely to promote greater food intake during the morning.

Breakfasts of Champions

Now that you know what breakfast should consist of, what should you eat? Use the suggestions below to fuel your days and get them off to the right start.

● 1 cup of yogurt and a piece of fruit.

● 1 cup of cereal, 1/2 cup of nonfat milk and 1/2 of a medium banana, sliced. Cereal should be whole-grain or 3 or more grams of fiber and less than 10 grams of sugar.

● Breakfast burrito: 4 egg whites, scrambled, 1 oz. of low-fat cheese, 1/4 cup of salsa and a whole-wheat tortilla.

● 1/2 cup of oatmeal and 8 oz. of orange juice.

● 1 whole-wheat English muffin and 2 Tbsp. low-fat ricotta cheese.

● 1 slice of whole-wheat or spelt bread, 1 Tbsp. of natural peanut butter and a small apple.

● A small nonfat milk or soy milk latte with a piece of fruit, like an apple or grapefruit.

● A smoothie made with 1 cup nonfat milk and 1 cup of frozen berries of your choice.

● 1 medium-size whole-wheat or rye bagel with 1 Tbsp. of light cream cheese.

● 1 small whole-wheat or rye bagel with 1 Tbsp. of light cream cheese and 2 oz. smoked salmon.

● Omelet made with 4 egg whites scrambled or 1 cup of EggBeaters mixed with 1/2 cup of spinach, mushrooms or any vegetable of your choice and an ounce of low-fat cheese.

● 1 cup of fat-free yogurt, 2 Tbsp. of granola and 1/4 cup of blueberries.

● 2 oz. of cheese, sliced, one small apple, sliced and 5 whole-grain crackers.

● 1 English muffin topped with 2 oz. of

shredded low-fat cheese and sliced apples baked at 400° F until cheese melts.

● 1 cup of bran flakes with 1/2 cup of non-fat milk and an 8-oz. glass of orange juice.

● A smoothie made with 1 cup of orange juice, a scoop of protein powder and 1/4 cup of mixed frozen berries.

Sample Week 5 Rise and Shine Goals:
This week, I will eat breakfast every day even if it's only a piece of fruit and a glass of milk.
or
This week, I will eat breakfast within one-half hour of waking up. I will record whether I am hungry or not in my food journal and eat accordingly.

Week 5 Rise and Shine Goals:

_____

_____

_____

_____

_____

_____

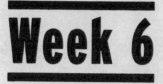

Week 6

Live a More Active Life

During a recent trip to Disneyland, I couldn't help but notice all of the overweight people — children and adults. These families were spending the summer day walking around and standing. But one day at the Magic Kingdom was not going to make them magically thinner or healthier. This day of moving would need to be a constant in their lives. When they returned home from their family vacations, how would they continue to move? I wondered.

A recent study found that modern Amish people have less than a 10 percent rate of obesity. These people do not rely on modern technologies to get their food, send mail or get from place to place. Most are not stuck at desk jobs. Instead, they are out in the fields pushing plows. Researchers found that the Amish diets had a relatively high amount of fat and were actually high in calories. The difference is that they are *moving*.

For the most part, we don't move. We are desk jockeys — stuck behind the computer where the only movement happening is your fingers traveling up and down the keyboard. The last time I checked, fingers were not a major muscle group; therefore, there aren't any heart-healthy benefits or serious calorie-burning happening right now. Where generations before us had to walk to the store to buy groceries or farm food or had jobs that were physical in nature, we have become sedentary with technology.

The hardest part is consciously moving. While you can workout and exercise, a healthy life begins with an active life. Think about your life — are you immersed in car culture? Do you walk to deliver memos or send them interoffice mail or by e-mail? Do you spend your free time playing with your pets and/or children? Do you prefer the stairs to the elevator? Adding these things to your life can make your everyday activities active.

10,000 Steps

Think about your typical day. How many steps do you think you take? According to the organization Shape Up America, the average person takes between 300 and 3,000 steps a day. To maintain weight, it's recommended that we get 30 minutes of exercise each day beyond our normal daily activities. In total, this would be about 10,000 steps a day. That may sound difficult to do if your day resembles the following: Get up and get ready for your day by walking back and forth between the bathroom and your closet. (If your house is newer, these things might be in the same room.) Go to the kitchen and make breakfast for you and possibly your children. Walk to family members' rooms to wake them up. Get everyone ready for school and work. Walk to the car, drive to work and walk from the parking lot to your desk. Park yourself at your desk until lunch or until you have to go to the bathroom. Walk from car to lunch spot. Return to your desk after lunch and get up only for bathroom breaks until it's time to go home. Get back into the car and pick up children from any daycare or after-school programs. Get home and make dinner. Help the kids with their homework. Sit on the couch and watch TV. Go to bed.

Not much movement. The thought of trying to exercise for 30 minutes may sound daunting but if you make a few changes to your everyday routine, you can take 10,000 steps a day. In the example above, just by adding the changes below, you can add quite a few steps. Be forewarned, these things do add time to your already busy day. But the time you take will help you immensely by clearing your mind, connecting with others and decreasing your stress levels.

In the morning, walk your children to their bus stop or to school. If you don't have children but have a pet, take it for a walk or play with it. When you park at your office, park as far as you can from the entrance as safely as possible. For your bathroom breaks during the day, go to a facility that is at the other end of the building or on a different floor (use the stairs). At lunch, take a walk

— five to 10 minutes is all you need. Do the same thing in the afternoon when you are starting to get sleepy. Play with your pet or children when you return home from work. And finally, after dinner, have the family go for a walk. Catch up on the day by walking and talking. These are only small additions to a day that you are already going through. Below are more suggestions to help you take 10,000 steps a day:

- Walk to the store to buy the ingredients for dinner.
- Take the stairs instead of the elevator.
- Meet a friend for a walk instead of a meal.
- Dance in your living room during commercials.
- For dessert, walk to your local ice cream parlor or grocery store.
- Take two- to three-minute walking breaks at work a few times a day.
- Change the TV channel manually. (Gasp!)
- March in place during TV commercials.
- Sit in a rocking chair and push off the floor with your feet.
- Do chores like lawn mowing, leaf raking, gardening and housework.
- Park farther away from entrances.

Have Fun With Your Free Time

Your time away from work and the pressures of your life can be your sanctuary. While sleeping in and being lazy is welcome, turning your free time into fun time is another way to lead an active lifestyle. Finding activities that you like to do can lead to stress reduction and the possibility of meeting people who enjoy the same things as you do. Signing up for tennis lessons, a softball league or a dance class can transport you to another place — mentally and physically. Also, what better excuse to leave the office on time? You can't let down the team.

If you have difficulty choosing an activity, look no further than your childhood. Did you play soccer? Maybe you were the roller-skating disco queen. Whatever the activity you enjoyed as a child, put it at the top of your list of things to try. If you find that you don't get the same enjoyment as you did when you were 10 years old, no problem — try something new. Maybe that Pilates studio down the street from your office has piqued your interest or maybe that tae kwon do dojo is calling your name. Whatever the activity, just do it. Since our culture is more sedentary in general, it takes more effort to move every day. That's why it is important to go out and find activities you enjoy.

Now Go Out and Have Fun!

Since losing weight is a numbers game based on input and output, I have crunched the numbers so that you can see how many calories you are burning during an hour of everyday activities.

If you do any of the activities listed in the chart on the next two pages for less time, just divide the number of minutes by 60 and multiply the outcome by the number of calories listed closest to your weight to find out approximately how many calories you burned.

For example, let's say you're 145 pounds and you were shopping for 45 minutes. To find the amount of calories burned: 45 minutes/60 minutes = 0.75 x 232 = 174 calories burned.

WEIGHT	100	105	110	115	120	125	130	135	140
Calories burned in 60 minutes									
Eating	72	76	79	83	86	90	94	97	101
Standing quietly	61	64	67	71	74	77	80	83	86
Weeding in the garden	216	227	238	248	259	270	281	292	302
Shopping (walking 2 mph)	160	168	176	184	192	200	208	216	224
Office work/ light cleaning	160	168	176	184	192	200	208	216	224
Disco dancing	228	239	251	262	274	285	296	308	319

145	150	155	160	165	170	175	180	185	190	195	200
104	108	112	115	119	122	126	130	133	137	140	144
89	92	95	98	101	104	107	110	113	117	120	123
313	324	335	346	356	367	378	389	400	410	421	432
232	240	248	256	264	272	280	288	296	304	312	320
232	240	248	256	264	272	280	288	296	304	312	320
331	342	353	365	376	388	399	410	422	433	445	456

This table was created with the formula from *Exercise and Your Heart — A guide to physical activity*. National Heart, Lung and Blood Institute/American Heart Association, DHHS, PHS, NIH Publication No. 93-1677.

Sample Week 6 Live a More Active Life Goals:

This week, I will try one new activity after work.

or

At least three times this week I will go for a walk with my family after dinner.

or

For my coffee break at work, I will go for a 10-minute walk.

Your Week 6 Live a More Active Life Goals:

_____

_____

_____

_____

_____

_____

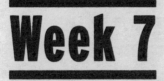

Deciphering Nutritional Labels

*L*earning more about food labels is an important step you can't skip when you are on a mission to eat right. This chapter will help pick apart the portions of the "Nutrition Facts" label on the side of most boxes. Ultimately, you shouldn't need to live or die by the nutritional labels but understanding them will help you make better food choices. You will be able to see that a little label knowledge will go a long way. I suggest that

you go to your kitchen cupboard right now
and grab a cereal box or other food item that
has an easy-to-read Nutrition Facts label.
Consider it a visual aid for this chapter.

Serving Size and Calories

I discuss this in detail in the portion size
chapter but here I will address it as it
relates to the label that you hold in your
hand. Calories provide a measure of how
much energy you get from a serving of this
food. The label also tells you how many of
the calories in one serving come from fat.

The U.S. Food and Drug Administration
says serving sizes listed on food labels are
meant to reflect the amount of the food
that you actually consume. This is rarely
the case. Think about it, do you eat that one
ounce of chips or that half-cup of cereal
that are the serving sizes? Probably not;
most of us don't. In fact, most of us consume more. This isn't necessarily a bad
thing. Think of the serving size as being
the measurement of servings that fit into
your food pyramid. It may not be the first
thing you look at when reading a food label,
but after determining how much you will

actually eat of the product, it will help provide useful information to determine how much fat, sugar, protein, carbohydrates and other nutrients you are consuming. It will also provide some insight when you are comparing similar products. For example, if you are comparing cereal, a serving size of Special K is 1 cup while a serving size of Fruity Pebbles is 1/2 cup. Both are 110 calories. (OK, now we know what is in my cupboard.) You get to eat more Special K for the same amount of calories that are in the Fruity Pebbles and you will probably feel fuller afterward.

How Many Calories Do You Need?

Eating too many calories per day is linked to excessive weight and obesity. But how are you supposed to know how many calories you should be eating? "There is no formula in the scientific literature that can help you definitely figure it out," says Walter Thompson, Ph.D., FACSM, FAACVPR, professor of kinesiology & health and professor of nutrition at Georgia State University in Atlanta. "A better estimate of the number of calories you should consume is to monitor your body weight. If you are weight-stable (that is, if your body weight does not fluctuate), calculate (or have a nutritionist calculate) the average number of calories you are now consuming. If you are weight-stable, then the number of calories you are consuming is equal to the number of calories you are expending."

Nutritionists generally will take a three-day average. If you are losing weight, the number of calories you are consuming is less than you're expending and if you are gaining weight, the number of calories you are consuming is greater than what you are expending. If you are already engaged in a strength-training program and as a result are increasing muscle mass (and not losing weight), your caloric intake is already at a sufficient level. Monitor your body weight and then determine if you need to increase your caloric consumption.

By the way, when you consume the additional calories needed to maintain body weight, you are already consuming the additional protein needed to increase muscle mass. There is no need to supplement your diet with more protein.

If you are satisfied with your current body weight and you aren't gaining or losing weight, your caloric consumption is just about right. Don't eat any more or any less. Weigh yourself once a week or so to check your weight loss or gain, then adjust your caloric consumption to match your need. There is no need to increase your caloric consumption, even if you change your goals. Simply monitor your body weight then increase or decrease your caloric consumption to match your new need for calories.

Total Fat

This line may catch your attention at first but do you know how to really read it? Unsaturated fat is a actually a "good" fat, because it can help lower LDL (bad) cholesterol and raise HDL (good) cholesterol.

Saturated Fats. "Bad" fat is the LDL cholesterol-raising saturated fat found in foods that are typically of animal origin, such as milk, meat and sour cream. You want to stay clear of foods that contain more than one-third saturated fat. These fats contribute to heart disease and some cancers, so you will want to make sure that saturated fats do not exceed 10 percent of your total caloric intake. Trans fat is also included under the saturated fat umbrella. Just recently the FDA has ruled that trans fats are to be listed on the "Nutrition Facts" label. Trans fat occurs naturally in some foods but is also produced when fats are hydrogenated — a process that makes oil solid by altering chemical states and creating fatty acids.

Until trans fats make their appearance on food labels, you can estimate the amount of trans fat in an item when saturated and unsaturated fats are listed. If you subtract the sum of the saturated and unsaturated fats from the number of total fat grams, you will get the amount of trans fat in the food product. This should be included in the 10 percent total of "bad" fat that makes up your total caloric intake.

Unsaturated Fats. Found most often in vegetable oils, unsaturated fats come in either the polyunsaturated or the monounsaturated variety and should constitute about 20 percent of your total daily caloric intake. Polyunsaturated fats are necessary for health and cannot be made by the body. Part of the omega-3 and omega-6 families, polyunsaturated fats can be found in fatty fish, such as salmon, mackerel and herring. It's thought to possibly help prevent heart disease because these fats lower triglycerides, reduce blood clotting, lower blood pressure and prevent irregular heartbeat. Monounsaturated fats are found in vegetable oils like olive, peanut and canola and are primarily consumed in Mediterranean-style diets.

How Much Fat Should You Have in Your Diet?

When deciding how much fat should be included in your diet, Thompson says: "According to the Federal Citizens Information Center, the Dietary Guidelines recommend that Americans limit fat in their diets to 30 percent of calories. This amounts to 53 grams of fat in a 1,600-calorie diet, 73 grams of fat in a 2,200-calorie diet and 93 grams of fat in a 2,800-calorie diet. You will get up to half this fat even if you pick the lowest fat choice from each good group and add no fat to your foods in preparation or at the table. You decide how to use the additional fat in your daily diet.

You may want to have foods from the five major food groups that are higher in fat — such as whole milk instead of skim. Or you may want to use it in cooking or at the table in the form of spreads, dressings or toppings. You don't need to count fat grams every day, but doing a fat checkup once in awhile will help keep you on the right track. If you find you are eating too much fat, choose lower-fat foods more often. You can figure the number of grams of fat that provide 30 percent of calories in your daily diet as follows:

Multiply your total day's calories by 0.30 to get your calories from fat per day. Example: 2,200 calories x 0.30 = 660 calories from fat.

Then,

Divide calories from fat per day by 9 (each gram of fat has 9 calories) to get grams of fat per day. Example: 660 calories from fat/9 = 73 grams of fat.

Cholesterol

Cholesterol is a tricky thing because we can get it from the foods we eat — butter, eggs and fatty meat — and our liver produces it. Excessive ingestion of foods containing cholesterol should be avoided because it contributes to heart disease.

The coronary arteries are prone to form plaque inside them. These plaques narrow the arterial vessels and in some people, the vessels become so narrow that blood can't be pumped through them. When the blood cannot be pumped to the heart, a person suffers a heart attack. It would seem that not eating cholesterol would help this. But certain diets signal the body to produce its own cholesterol.

Diets high in saturated fat stimulate cholesterol production by the liver, raising its levels in the blood. These fats are most abundant in fatty red meats, butter and some milk products. On the other hand, evidence exists that polyunsaturated or monounsaturated fats such as olive oil and corn oil do not promote cholesterol production.

Sodium and Potassium

Though we try to keep our sodium intake to a minimum because it can raise blood pressure and contribute to hypertension, we actually need it in certain foods like sports drinks. That's because if you are exercising heavily, your body loses sodium and potassium in sweat. Sodium is also necessary to keep foods flavorful and preserved. Your intake shouldn't exceed 2,400 milligrams per day. (Contact your doctor to determine whether this is a good benchmark for you.)

Total Carbohydrate

The typical American diet consists of 40 percent to 60 percent of its calories in carbohydrates. Sugars and fiber are both carbohydrates and are covered in great detail in other areas of this book. Over the years, our consumption of simple sugars like high fructose syrup has risen and constitute a large portion of our carbohydrate intake. While simple sugars occur naturally in fruits, vegetables and dairy products, sugars are also present in food items like soups, spaghetti sauce, cereals, yogurt, fruit drinks, frozen dinners, condiments such as ketchup and much more. Cookies, candies, cakes and white bread consist predominantly of carbohydrates.

In the body, carbohydrates are the predominant energy source filling the muscles to fuel their movements. During digestion, carbohydrate molecules are absorbed into the bloodstream to individual cells. Inside the cell, glucose, the most common form of carbohydrate, is transformed into glycogen or used directly for energy. Once the glycogen stores are full, any extra carbohydrate that has been eaten is synthesized into fat. This explains how body fat increases by eating too many carbohydrates. But don't let this deter you.

Carbohydrates must be eaten on a regular basis to maintain the body's glycogen stores. If the levels get too low, the "back-up" glycogen is tapped into. And carbohydrate isn't just an energy fuel. It helps maintain tissue protein. When glycogen stores are reduced, your body starts to convert glucose from protein. This results in a reduction of lean muscle mass, which eventually slows your metabolism and burdens the kidneys as they excrete the nitrogen-containing byproducts of protein breakdown.

Protein

With the popularity of low-carb diets and the Atkins Revolution, Americans tend to get more than enough protein. The amount of protein you need differs from person to person and that's why there isn't a percentage of daily intake listed on the food label. Scientific studies suggest that protein intake for those who engage in regular, intense strength-building exercise should be 0.7 to 0.8 grams of protein per pound of body weight; those who engage in active exertion on a regular basis should be consuming 0.5 to 0.6 grams of protein per pound of body weight, and sedentary individuals should be consuming 0.4 grams of protein per pound of body weight.

Use the chart on the facing page to figure out your protein needs based on your activity level and weight.

Grams of Protein Per Pound Based On Energy Level

Weight	Activity levels		
	Sedentary or sporadic exerciser	Active exerciser	Very active – weightlifters & endurance athletes
110	44	66	88
120	48	72	96
130	52	78	104
140	56	84	112
150	60	90	120
160	64	96	128
170	68	102	136
180	72	108	144
190	76	114	152
200	80	120	160
210	84	126	168
220	88	132	176

Vitamins and Minerals

Just after protein is a list of vitamins and their percentage of daily intake value. These vitamins have value in your diet by helping your body function properly. Collectively, these make up your micronutrients. Alone, they do not supply you with energy but they aid important bodily functions. Below and on the following pages, you will find a list of common vitamins and their functions.

Vitamin	Daily Intake	Function(s)
B1 or Thiamine	1.1-1.4 mg	• Aids carbohydrate metabolism. • Required for proper muscle and nerve function. • Helps regulate appetite.
B2 or Riboflavin	1.1-1.4 mg	• Aids carbohydrate and protein metabolism.

Vitamin	Daily Intake	Function(s)
		● Promotes tissue repair. ● Helps body use oxygen. ● Aids in good vision.
B3 or Niacin	16-18 mg	● Essential for energy releasing reactions and cell metabolism. ● Aids carbohydrate metabolism. ● Supports healthy skin, nervous system and digestive system.
B6 or Pyridoxine	1.3-2.0 mg	● Required for normal metabolism of amino acids and fats. ● Helps produce red blood cells.

Vitamin	Daily Intake	Function(s)
B12 or Cyanocobalamin	2.4-2.6 mg	● Required for red blood cell formation and proper function of nervous system. ● Helps break down some fatty acids.
Pantothenic acid	5-6 mg	● Helps convert metabolic fuels into energy. ● Required for normal nerve and immune function.
Biotin	25-20 mg	● Aids fatty acid synthesis. ● Helps carbohydrate and amino acid metabolism. ● Needed for maintaining healthy skin.

Vitamin	Daily Intake	Function(s)
Folic acid	400-600 mcg	● Coenzyme for some metabolic processes. ● Required for red blood cell production.
C or Ascorbic acid	1,000 mg	● Essential for strong teeth and bones and tissue healing. ● Aids the absorption of iron. ● Aids in collagen and thyroxin synthesis. ● It is an antioxidant. ● Helps maintain immune system. ● Aids amino acid synthesis.

Vitamin	Daily Intake	Function(s)
A or Retinol	5,000 IU	● Needed for good night vision. ● Helps maintain skin. ● Maintenance of cornea and tooth and bone growth. ● Aids reproduction. ● Aids immune system. ● *Dosages far in excess of the maximum daily requirement have been known to cause illness, as a result of long-term overuse.*
D or Calciferol	200-400 IU	● Needed for calcium and phosphorous metabolism.

Vitamin	Daily Intake	Function(s)
		● Aids bone growth and mineralization of bone tissue. *● Dosages far in excess of the maximum daily requirement may cause illness, as a result of long-term overuse.*
E or Tocopherol	30 IU	● It is an antioxidant. ● Inhibits catabolism of fatty acids in cell membrane. ● Protects vitamin A.
K	60-80 mcg	● Needed for normal blood clotting. ● Helps regulate blood calcium levels.

Mineral	Daily Intake	Function(s)
Iron	18 mg	● Major component of protein hemoglobin (carries oxygen) and myoglobin (aids in muscle contraction). ● *Dosages far in excess of the maximum daily requirement for iron have been known to cause illness, as a result of long-term overuse.*
Calcium	1,000-1,300 mg	● Bone formation. ● Maintenance of healthy bones. ● Muscular contraction and relaxation. ● Nerve function.

Mineral	Daily Intake	Function(s)
		● Blood clotting. ● Blood pressure regulation. ● Immune defenses.
Potassium	2,000 mg	● Maintain fluid and electrolyte balance. ● Supports cell integrity. ● Aids muscle contractions. ● Helps nerve impulse transmission. ● *Dosages far in excess of the maximum daily requirement for potassium have been known to cause illness, as a result of long-term overuse.*

Mineral	Daily Intake	Function(s)
Phosphorous	0.7-1.25 g	● Aids bone formation. ● It is part of every cell as part of RNA, DNA and phospholipids. ● Aids acid balance. ● Aids energy transfer. ● *Dosages far in excess of the maximum daily requirement for phosphorous have been known to cause illness, as a result of long-term overuse.*
Iodine	150 mcg	● Regulates growth, development and metabolism.

Mineral	Daily Intake	Function(s)
		● *Dosages far in excess of the maximum daily requirement for iodine have been known to cause illness, as a result of long-term overuse.*
Magnesium	310-420 mcg	● Helps bone mineralization. ● Builds proteins. ● Helps enzyme action and muscle contraction. ● Aids nerve impulse transmission. ● Aids immune system. ● *Dosages far in excess of the maximum daily*

Mineral	Daily Intake	Function(s)
		requirement for magnesium have been known to cause illness, as a result of long-term overuse.
Zinc	15 mg	● Makes RNA and DNA. ● Supports immune function. ● Helps transport vitamin A. ● Aids wound healing. ● Helps taste perception. ● Aids sperm production and fetus development. ● Helps insulin production. ● *Dosages far*

Mineral	Daily Intake	Function(s)
		in excess of the maximum daily requirement for zinc have been known to cause illness, as a result of long-term overuse.
Chloride	750 mg	● Maintains fluid and electrolyte balance. ● Aids in proper digestion. ● *Dosages far in excess of the maximum daily requirement for chloride have been known to cause illness, as a result of long-term overuse.*

Mineral	Daily Intake	Function(s)
Sodium	500 mg	● Maintains fluid and electrolyte balance. ● Aids nerve impulse transmission. ● Helps muscle contraction. ● *Dosages far in excess of the maximum daily requirement for sodium have been known to cause illness, as a result of long-term overuse.*
Selenium	55-70 mcg	● Works with vitamin E as an antioxidant. ● *Dosages far in excess of the the maximum daily*

Mineral	Daily Intake	Function(s)
		requirement for selenium have been known to cause illness, as a result of long-term overuse.
Copper	2 mg	● Aids absorption and use of iron. ● Is part of many enzymes. ● *Dosages far in excess of the maximum daily requirement for copper have been known to cause illness, as a result of long-term overuse.*
Manganese	2-5 mg	● Facilitator of many cell processes.

Mineral	Daily Intake	Function(s)
		● *Dosages far in excess of the maximum daily requirement for manganese have been known to cause illness, as a result of long-term overuse.*
Fluoride	2.9-3.8 mg	● Aids in formation of teeth and bones. ● *Dosages far in excess of the maximum daily requirement for fluoride have been known to cause illness, as a result of long-term overuse.*
Chromium	50-200 mcg	● Helps release energy from glucose.

Mineral	Daily Intake	Function(s)
		● *Dosages far in excess of the maximum daily requirement for chromium have been known to cause illness, as a result of long-term overuse.*
Molybdenum	75-250 mcg	● Facilitator of many cell processes.
		● *Dosages far in excess of the maximum daily requirement for molybdenum have been known to cause illness, as a result of long-term overuse.*

mg=milligrams (1/1,000 of a gram)
mcg=micrograms (1/1,000,000 of a gram)
IU=International Units of measurement

Understanding the Ingredients

Scanning an ingredient list can be mind-numbing, but if you know what to look for, you'll be able to determine what you're really getting. The cardinal rule of the ingredient list is that order matters because they are listed by weight — most to least prevalent. Sugar and items that you cannot pronounce or cannot easily identify are not great things to be listed first. A shorter list is better because the ingredients are probably natural.

The Percent Daily Value (%DV)

This part of the Nutrition Facts panel tells you whether the nutrients (fat, sodium, fiber, etc.) in a serving of food contribute a lot or a little to your total daily diet. The percent daily values (%DV) are based on recommendations for a 2,000- calorie diet. For labeling purposes, the FDA set 2,000 calories as the reference amount for calculating Percent Daily Values. This number shows you the percentage (or how much) of the recommended daily amount of a nutrient is in a serving of food. By using the

%DV, you can tell if this amount is high or low. You, like most people, may not know how many calories you consume in a day. But you can still use the %DV as a frame of reference, whether or not you eat more or less than 2,000 calories each day.

Likewise, you should try to get enough essential nutrients, such as calcium, iron and vitamins A and C, as well as other components such as dietary fiber. Try to average 100 percent for each one of these nutrients each day.

Label Lingo

Food producers are marketers. And when you are standing in the aisles of the grocery store scanning the shelves to decide what cereal, bread, cookie, salad dressing, etc. that you are going to put in your cart and take home, the information overload is just plain overwhelming. Besides the Nutrition Facts label, food makers try to lure you with package labeling that they hope will catch your eye and help you make that purchasing decision. Use the chart on the following pages to decipher the seals, certifications and health claims that can cloud your good sense.

Label	What It Means
American Heart Association Mark of Approval	The product meets the criteria for heart-healthy levels of fat (less than or equal to 3 grams), saturated fat (less than or equal to 1 gram), cholesterol (less than or equal to 20 milligrams), sodium (less than or equal to 480 milligrams) and provides at least 10 %DV of protein, vitamin A, vitamin C, calcium, iron or dietary fiber.
No artificial flavoring	The product contains only flavors that occur naturally in foods. There are roughly 2,000 flavoring agents that are allowed in foods. The most common is MSG or Accent.
No artificial coloring	The product does not contain any of the coloring agents that are allowed in foods. Naturally occurring colors come from carrot oils, grape skin or beet juice.
Low-calorie, diet or reduced-calorie	The product contains no more than 40 calories in a single serving or a maximum of 0.4 calories per gram, or one-third

Label	What It Means
	fewer calories than the regular product.
Cholesterol-free	The product contains less than 2 mg of cholesterol per serving.
No Cholesterol	The product does not contain any cholesterol.
Enriched	Vitamins (riboflavin, niacin and thiamine) and the mineral iron have been added to the product because it originally lacked them or they were destroyed during processing.
Fat-free	The product contains less than 0.5 grams of fat per serving.
Low-fat	If it is on a package of meat, the fat content does not exceed 10% fat by weight. If it is on a package of milk, the fat content can range from 0.5 to 2%.
Fortified	Vitamins and minerals have been added because the product did not contain them before.
Fresh Frozen	Food was quickly frozen while still fresh.

Label	What It Means
More, Added, Extra or Plus	10% or more of the daily value of each referenced amount. May only be used for vitamins, minerals, protein, dietary fiber and potassium.
Good Source of, Contains or Provides	10%-19% of the daily value of the referenced amount. These terms may be used on meals or main dishes to indicate that product contains a food that meets definition. May not be used for total carbohydrate.
High, Rich In or Excellent Source Of	Contains 20% or more of the daily value to describe protein, vitamins, minerals, dietary fiber or potassium. May be used on meals or main dishes to indicate that product contains a food that meets definition. May not be used for total carbohydrate.
Extra Lean	On seafood or poultry that contains less than 5 grams total fat, less than 2 grams saturated fat and less than 95 milligrams cholesterol per serving and per 100 grams. Meals and main dishes

Label	What It Means
	must meet per 100 grams and per labeled serving criteria.
Lean	On seafood or poultry that contains less than 10 grams total fat, 4.5 grams or less saturated fat and less than 95 milligrams cholesterol per serving and per 100 grams. Meals and main dishes must meet per 100 grams and per labeled serving criteria.
Light or Lite	● A food representative of the type of food bearing the claim (e.g., average value of top three brands). ● Similar food (e.g., potato chips for potato chips). ● And not low-calorie and low-fat (except light-sodium foods which must be low-calorie and low-fat).
Reduced and Added (or Fortified and Enriched)	The value of the referenced item is in comparison to an established regular product or average representative product and it is a similar food.

Label	What It Means
More and Less (or Fewer)	The value of the referenced item is in comparison to an established regular product and a dissimilar food in the same product category which may be generally substituted for the labeled food (e.g., potato chips for pretzels) or a similar food.
Imitation	The product has been changed from the original recipe by adding a substance. This is sometimes done to reduce its caloric content. Therefore, it only resembles or is a substitute for the product but it is nutritionally inferior to the food it imitates.
Natural	The product is as it occurs in nature, without additives, preservatives and artificial coloring or flavoring.
USDA-Organic	The product was grown without pesticides or growth hormones. Produce is farmed with environmental-friendly techniques. Livestock feed

Label	What It Means
	is free of animal proteins. For milk, cows are not treated with antibiotics.
Wheat	This product contains wheat but not necessarily whole-wheat. Check the ingredients label.
Sodium-free	This product contains less than 5 milligrams of sodium per serving.
Low-sodium	This product contains no more than 140 milligrams of sodium per serving.
Very-low-sodium	This product contains no more than 35 milligrams of sodium per serving.

Sample Week 7 Nutrition Facts Goals:

This week, I will read all the food labels on my favorite foods and decide whether they are good or bad for me.

or

When I go grocery shopping this week, I will buy one item that has 3 grams of fiber, one item that has 200 calories or less per serving and one item that comes in a single-serving package.

Your Week 7 Nutrition Facts Goals:

_____

_____

_____

_____

_____

_____

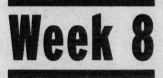

Portioning It Out

As food portions in this country increased, so did the size of the average American. Coupled with a sedentary lifestyle, our increased calorie count has had nowhere to go but to our thighs, hips and bellies. Our total calorie intake has increased approximately 200 calories a day since the late 1970s. The reason? The increase of portion sizes that occurred at that time. There is scientific evidence that suggests this direct relationship of portion size and intake is formed as young as age 3. It is this environmental factor which precedes our physiological hunger needs that help dictate the balance of energy being consumed in the form of food and of energy being expelled in the form of movement.

While we should take the blame upon ourselves, it is hard not to feel duped. For the longest time, a can of soda was considered two servings. Shouldn't that one hand-held can that is difficult to keep the leftovers in be considered one serving? It is now; one 250-calorie serving. But, when you buy snack sizes or go to a restaurant, you would like to think that those portions are considered one serving. That isn't the case. Look at these examples from the American Institute for Cancer Research:

● The croissant in France has a circumference of 15 inches and contains 174 calories and 11 grams of fat on average; in the United States, the circumference is 18 inches, with 270 calories and 15 grams of fat.

● When Jewish bakers introduced the bagel to the United States, it weighed 1.5 ounces and contained 116 calories. Today the bagel weighs 4.5 ounces and contains 350 to 400 calories on average.

● In Mexico, the quesadilla is cooked in a 5-inch corn tortilla and contains 540 calories and 32 grams of fat on the average. The same item made in American restaurant chains is a 10-inch flour tortilla and yields 1,200 calories and 70 grams of fat on average.

Source: American Institute for Cancer Research. When foreign foods are Americanized: Everything gets bigger stateside — including Americans. Available: http://www.AICR.org/press.

Looking at these examples it is easy to see how your portion expectations have become skewed. After seeing restaurant portions, when you are cooking your own meals they can look pretty puny.

In the battle of weight management, the primary strategy should be perfecting the portion size. This will help keep the balance of calories in tact without counting calories. This chapter will teach you how to learn portion control by sectioning your plate and learning portion sizes for food.

Perfecting the Plate

By just looking at your plate, you can start portioning your meals.

First, divide your plate into fourths:
- 1/4 of your plate is for starchy carbohydrates: potatoes, yams, whole-grain bread, beans;
- 1/4 of your plate is for protein: chicken, fish, beef or pork,
- and the last 1/2 of your plate is reserved for fruits and vegetables.

This becomes your starting plate. As you fill your plate, notice how your body responds to the foods you are eating. It might be that you feel sluggish after eating so many starchy carbohydrates; if so, replace with more vegetables or fruit.

Another version of this is "The New American Plate" designed by the American Institute for Cancer Research. This plate consists of two-thirds (or more) of vegetables, fruits, whole grains and beans and one-third (or less) of animal protein. It's intended to help people shift from a meat-centered meal to a predominantly plant-based meal without counting calories. As you become familiar with portion sizes, you may want to change the size of your plate from a dinner-size plate to a salad plate. This size change alone will change your perception of the amount of food you are eating.

Since everyone is chemically different, our plates will look different. And as we continue through this book, we will talk more about food choices so that you can create the healthiest plate possible for you.

Size Matters

There is nothing standard in serving sizes. Now, if an item is to be consumed in one sitting, it is considered a single serving. The standard serving size found on every can or jar are those of the U.S. Department of Agriculture. On the next two pages, you will find them listed and probably be shocked at how small they are.

Standard Serving Sizes

Food	Serving	Looks like
Chopped Vegetables	1/2 cup	1/2 baseball or rounded handful for the average adult.
Raw Leafy Vegetables (like lettuce)	1 cup	1 baseball or the fist of an average adult.
Fresh Fruit	1 medium fruit	1 tennis ball
Chopped	1/2 cup	1/2 baseball or rounded handful for the average adult.
Juice	3/4 cup (6 oz.)	Small glass
Dried Fruit	1/4 cup	1 golf ball or scant handful for the average adult.
Pasta, Rice, Cooked Cereal	1/2 cup	1/2 baseball or rounded handful for average adult.
Ready-to-Eat (dried) Cereal	1 oz., which varies from 1/2 cup to 1 1/4 cups (check label)	

Food	Serving	Looks like
Meat, Poultry, Seafood	3 oz. (boneless cooked weight from 4 oz. raw)	Deck of cards.
Dried Beans	1/2 cup cooked	1/2 baseball or rounded handful for average adult.
Nuts	1/3 cup	Level handful for an adult.
Peanut Butter	2 Tbsp.	1 golf ball.
Cheese	1 1/2 oz. (2 oz. if processed cheese)	1 oz. looks like 4 dice. 1 1/2 oz. is about 3 dominoes.

To learn these portions, do this exercise for each night's dinner for a week. Measure your usual portion size onto a plate or bowl. Make a mental note of how much of your plate is covered or your bowl is filled. After checking the chart above, measure a standard serving of the same food onto the same size plate or bowl. Compare. Ask yourself how many standard servings go into the portion you normally eat. If your weight is satisfactory, you are probably eating the right portions to balance the energy input and output. If you are overweight, the first thing you should consider is reducing the number of standard servings in your regular portion.

Serving Single

In the grand scheme of life, remember that you are not limited to one serving of food at a time and that our ideas of portion sizes have been distorted by America's super-sizing of everything from appetizers to dessert. Looking at one serving of some foods will make you feel some deprivation. But having said that, a single serving can be a key to weight loss. In fact, portion control is vital to weight loss. It is impossible to know how many calories are in the foods we eat, but limiting ourselves to one portion or a "single serving" is a great start and meal replacements may be the answer. In individual, prepackaged portions, meal replacements offer portion-controlled meals that are easy to prepare and may make your weight-loss plan much easier to follow.

The perfect example of a meal replacement is a can of Slim-Fast. It's a single serving item meant to replace a regular meal and contains carbohydrates, protein and fat. Meal replacements are typically portion-controlled prepackaged meals used in place of meals that are prepared from scratch. They are mostly in liquid form, but researchers like John Jakicic, Ph.D., of the Physical Activity and Weight Management Research Center at the University of Pittsburgh and others have expanded the category to include such items as nutrition bars, Lean Cuisine or Healthy Choice-type frozen entrees and certain kinds of canned soup. Depending how far you want to expand the category, Subway sandwiches are an example of a single serving and Jared Fogle's weight loss was no accident.

Meal replacements have been the subject of many weight-reduction studies. They have been shown to be an effective strategy for the long-term maintenance of weight loss as well as the promotion of greater short-term weight loss compared with traditional calorie-reduction strategies. So why does it work?

You are essentially preventing yourself from overeating. You are eating food that you would normally be eating anyway, except that you are using a prepackaged concept to limit its fat and calories. So consider potato chips part of the program. Eaten in a single-serving snack size, it's much easier to eat only one — serving that is.

Sometimes it's just impossible to know how many calories you are eating, especially if you eat in restaurants often, because you have no idea how your food was prepared. Meal replacements are defined products so you know exactly how many calories they have. There isn't any guesswork when it comes to the composition of the meal, the size of the meal or anything like that. And just like restaurants, the convenience of a meal replacement makes it a lucrative way to watch your portion sizes without skipping meals.

If you decide to take on a single-serving plan, realize that you will be able to spot overeating more easily than when you are eating other foods. For example, if you are eating cereal, it's simple to unconsciously pour more into the bowl or go back for seconds when you are dealing with a big box. If you are using those single-serving packets that you used to have at camp or in your school cafeteria, you will have to physically open another box to have another helping of cereal. It may even get your attention long enough for you to rethink that second serving.

As another bonus for people who have gastrointestinal problems is that while shakes and bars can wreak havoc on your system, incorporating frozen meals, soups and sandwiches becomes a more palatable option. For weight management, Jakicic recommends substituting a meal replacement for one or two regular meals a day. Here are some tips on how to do this:

● Eat a meal replacement for one or two meals per day — a shake, bar, frozen entree or can of soup that contains one serving per package. Each product should contain 200 to 400 calories.

● Eat at least one traditional healthy meal containing fresh foods each day. It should include a minimum of one serving of fruits and vegetables and one serving of whole grains. You don't want that one traditional meal to come from the drive-thru at McDonald's.

● Use the meal replacement for a meal that you consider a fuel stop. By this I mean, don't break out the meal replacement for a meal when the experience is most of the meal — dinner with the family or lunch with friends. Breakfast is a good candidate if it's eaten alone or on the run. Lunch at your desk becomes an easy meal replacement situation because you can pop a frozen entrée into the lunchroom microwave.

● Eat snacks of fruits and vegetables. Meal replacements tend to lack fiber, phytochemicals and other nutrients so it is important to augment your diet with these healthful offerings.

● Vary your meal replacement intake. Eating the same thing can get boring so alternate the varieties and types of food.

● Consider using meal replacements for one or two meals on the weekdays then take a break over the weekend.

A Sample Single-Serving Day

Breakfast	• A packet of ready-to-eat oatmeal • 1/2 cup of fat-free milk • 1/2 of a medium grapefruit
Snack	• 6 oz. low-fat yogurt sprinkled with 1 Tbsp. wheat germ
Lunch	• 1 (9.75-oz.) Lean Cuisine Café Classics Roasted Turkey Breast entrée
Snack	• 12 baby carrots • 1 single serving bag of whole-wheat pretzels
Dinner	• 1 grilled chicken breast, 1 cup of steamed broccoli and 1 cup of cooked brown rice.

Examples of everyday single servings

Grains (80 to 100 calories per serving)
- 1/2 cup cooked oats
- 1 mini bagel
- 1/2 cup cooked pasta
- 1 slice of bread
- 1/2 cup of cooked rice
- 1 cup Cheerios (1 ounce)
- 1/2 cup Total cereal (1 ounce)
- 1 Nature Valley granola bar
- 5 Triscuits
- 1/2 regular bagel, English muffin, bun or pita

Lean Protein (100 calories/serving)
- 6 egg whites
- 8 ounces fat-free milk (or 1% milk)
- 1 piece of string cheese
- 3 ounces canned tuna packed in water
- 3 ounces lean ground turkey
- 6 ounces light yogurt
- 3 ounces turkey or chicken breast
- 2/3 cup cottage cheese (low-fat or fat-free)

Fruit (60 calories per serving)
- 1/4 cup dried fruit
- 1/2 cup canned peaches in extra-light syrup
- 1 orange
- 8 ounces of 100% juice
- 1/2 cup grapefruit

Vegetables (25 calories per serving)
- 1/2 cup raw sliced or chopped vegetables
- 1 cup lettuce
- 1/2 cup beans
- 1/2 cup chopped cooked vegetables
- 1 small potato

Sample Week 8 Portioning It Out Goals:

I will eat at least six servings of grains, four servings of protein, three servings of fruits and vegetables each day this week.

or

I will eat at least four meals this week that are prepackaged single servings.

or

I will do the serving comparison exercise each night at dinner this week.

<u>Your Week 8 Portioning It Out Goals:</u>

_____

_____

_____

_____

_____

_____

_____

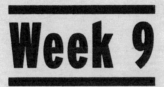

Eat More Fiber

*T*his week your goal is to try to eat more fiber. The American Cancer Society and the National Cancer Institute recommend eating 20 to 30 grams of fiber per day. This is most easily achieved by eating three to five servings of fruits and vegetables.

A serving is a half-cup of cooked or raw vegetables or one cup of leafy, raw salad vegetables; a serving of fruit consists of one medium apple, banana or orange, half a grapefruit, one melon wedge, three-quarters cup of juice, one-half cup of berries or one-quarter cup of dried fruit.

Whole grains and beans also provide fiber while animal protein (meat) contains none.

By adding fiber to your diet, you will feel fuller longer because fiber is resistant to human digestion. This helps fights fat, cholesterol and certain cancers. There are two types of fiber: soluble and insoluble.

Soluble fiber dissolves in water to become gummy or viscous. It also supports the growth of good intestinal bacteria and binds to cholesterol, thus helping to eliminate it and decreasing serum cholesterol levels. Oats and barley are types of soluble fiber.

Insoluble fiber holds water and helps move waste through the intestine quickly. Wheat is an example of an insoluble fiber. This is why a fiber-rich meal reduces the amount of calories that you absorb by binding to some of the fat you eat and preventing the fat's absorption. Fiber accelerates the food's movement through the body so fewer calories are available to the body.

Fiber-rich foods and meals also slow the breakdown and delay the absorption of glucose into your bloodstream, thereby lowering the food's glycemic effect; thus, leading to greater satiety after meals, as well as better blood sugar levels and appetite control between meals. Focusing on fiber-rich, low-glycemic foods at meals and snacks allows you to eat larger volumes of food and take in more nutrients without the excess calories.

Whole Grains: Superstar Fiber Source

The average American consumes between 0.8 to 1 servings of whole grains per day while the recommended amount of servings is three. If you are like most Americans, you have never eaten whole-grain bread, which is one of the easiest ways to consume whole grains.

Whole grains comprise three main layers: the bran, the endosperm and the germ. Even though grains are categorized as carbohydrates, they deliver much more than carbohydrate to our nutrient intake. While both whole and enriched grains are part of a healthy diet, you will see that when deciding between a whole-grain variety and an enriched variety, you will get more nutritional bang for your buck with whole grains.

One reason to include enriched foods in our diet is that since 1998 the United States has mandated that all flour products be fortified with folic acid in an attempt to limit birth defects. And this has been successful — since 2001, the amount of healthy births has increased.

Besides preventing birth defects, folic acid may also help prevent coronary disease and some cancers. The problem is that although refined grains have a role in a healthy diet, most Americans eat them exclusively and never touch a whole grain.

On the next page is a chart of the nutrient content of whole-meal flour and unfortified white flour per kilogram. It illustrates how the milling process concentrates the carbohydrate and reduces the concentrations of other macronutrients, vitamins and minerals due to the removal of the outer layers of the grain.

	Whole-meal flour	White flour
Protein (g)	127	94
Fat (g)	22	13
Carbohydrate (g)	639	777
Starch (g)	618	762
Sugars (g)	21	15
Fiber (g)	90	31
Sodium (mg)	30	30
Potassium (mg)	3,400	1,500
Calcium (mg)	380	150
Magnesium (mg)	1,200	200
Phosphorus (mg)	3,200	1,100
Iron (mg)	39	15
Copper (mg)	4.5	1.5
Zinc (mg)	29	6
Chloride (mg)	380	810
Manganese (mg)	31	6
Selenium (mg)	530	40
Vitamin E (mg)	14	3
Thiamine (mg)	4.7	1
Riboflavin (mg)	0.9	0.3
Niacin (mg)	57	7
Vitamin B6 (mg)	5	1.5
Folate	570	220

Adapted from Smith, A.T., Kuzenesof, S.,
Richardson, DP., Seal, C.J. Proceedings of the
Nutrition Society (2003), 62, 457.

Low consumption of whole grains is a major contributor to the lack of fiber in the American diet. American adults consume between 12 and 15 grams of fiber per day. This is woefully low compared to the 38 grams for men and the 25 grams for women per day that have been recommended as the most recent Dietary Reference Intakes by the National Academy of Sciences Macronutrient Report.

The American Heart Association, U.S. Dietary Guidelines and Healthy People 2010 recommended that consumers choose at least six daily servings of several grain products. In a nod to the importance of whole grains to the diet and recognizing the difficulty of adding whole grains to the diet because of taste and outside influences, Healthy People 2010 designates that three servings of whole grains should be included into a person's daily diet. (This is a recommendation that this book will help you strive to reach.)

Whole grains offer a unique nutrient package. In addition to vitamins and minerals, whole grains supply unsaturated fatty acids, tacotrienols, tocopherols, insoluble fiber, phytosterols, stanols, sphingolipids, phytates, lignins and numerous antioxidants.

When the bran and the germ of the grain are removed, 75 percent of the phytonutrients, along with the B vitamins, vitamin E, trace minerals and unsaturated fats, are lost. There goes the benefits.

Antioxidants are important anticarcinogenic agents due to their role in balancing oxidation and counteracting stress in the body. While we tend to consume fruits and vegetables to provide us with disease-fighting antioxidants, the truth is that the average antioxidant activity in whole-grain bread and cereals is at least equal to that of fruits and vegetables per serving.

In comparison to some berries, the antioxidant content of whole grains is less, but it is greater than that of common fruits or vegetables. Furthermore, some of the phytonutrients in whole grains are unique to grains and seeds and, therefore, cannot be obtained by eating only fruits and vegetables.

Fruits and Vegetables: The Plants Reign

Although fruits and vegetables are among the easiest ways to get fiber and other phytochemicals, consumption of these foods is still below the "five a day" mantra that has

been drilled into our heads. It may be that
we believe that we are eating more fruits
and vegetables than we truly are.
Researchers out of the Netherlands con-
ducted a study to determine if there was a
difference between people's intentions to
eat fruits and vegetables and misconcep-
tions about how many fruits and vegetables
they actually ate. What they found was a
prevalence of misconception about fruit
and vegetable consumption. Once the dis-
crepancy between actual and perceived was
pointed out, the study participants did
make an effort to consume more fruits and
vegetables in their diets.

Binding Benefits

There are so many wonderful things that
are included in whole grains and other plant
food and are associated with a reduced risk
for heart disease, stroke, certain cancers and
diabetes, as well as possibly being associated
with a lower incidence of obesity.

Heart Disease. There is much scientific
evidence linking the effects of whole grains
to heart health. All show a reduction of
coronary heart disease risk with whole-

grain consumption from anywhere between 25 percent to 35 percent. In fact, in a cohort of 34,000 Seventh-Day Adventists, those who preferred whole-grain bread over white bread had a lower risk of coronary disease. Similar results have been associated with cereal fiber and total fiber intakes.

Cancer. There is a 21 percent to 43 percent decrease in cancer risk associated with a diet high in whole-grain consumption. Possible mechanisms for the protective effects of whole grains against cancers include: alterations in carbohydrate fermentation, fecal bulk, transit time through the colon, endogenous sex hormone production, antioxidant activity and intestine and liver circulation.

Diabetes. Large-scale studies suggest that whole-grain consumption may have a preventive effect against diabetes. Researchers at the University of Minnesota (St. Paul) and the College of St. Catherine (St. Paul, Minnesota) have proposed that the greater the grain's particle size, less refining and high levels of soluble fiber in whole grains are associated with the lower glucose response that may help regulate blood sugar and lower the long-term risk of diabetes.

Cholesterol. Substitution of oat-based cereals for regular carbohydrate sources has been shown to reduce total cholesterol and LDL cholesterol (the bad kind). One study investigated the cholesterol-lowering effect of a ready-to-eat whole-grain-oat breakfast cereal in 124 males and females between the ages of 40 and 70 that had high cholesterol. The participants ate approximately 85 grams of oat breakfast cereal or corn-based breakfast cereal for six weeks. The group consuming the oat-based breakfast reduced their total cholesterol and LDL-cholesterol levels by 4 percent.

Obesity. While more studies are needed to verify the relationship between fiber consumption, whole-grain intake and weight-management, there has been an association between fiber intake and the prevalence to be overweight. In a study comparing normal, moderately obese and severely obese individuals in the United States, the normal individuals consumed 19 grams of fiber daily. In comparison, the obese individuals only consumed between 13 and 14 grams of fiber respectively. Theoretically, increasing whole-grain consumption is a useful dietary strategy to reduce the amount of calories in a person's diet, thereby aiding weight-loss efforts or minimizing weight gain.

Bulking Up

Getting the recommended 20 to 30 grams of fiber per day can be challenging. Use these tips and tricks to bulk up on this much-needed carbohydrate.

● Use the check-mark calendar at the end of this chapter. Place it on your refrigerator and mark your servings each day.

● Try a new vegetable and a new fruit each week.

● Eat three whole grains a day.

● Try to have at least one fruit or vegetable at each meal.

● Try familiar foods in new recipes, like adding beans to salads, casseroles and egg dishes.

● Make sure you drink at least eight glasses of water a day to help your body process all of this fiber more easily. If not, you may experience flatulence.

● Chew well, since fiber-rich foods need to be well-masticated to be digested properly.

● Focus on fresh and frozen, rather than canned, vegetables and fruits and use dried fruits in modest portions.

● Eat oatmeal, buckwheat pancakes or barley at breakfast. If you prefer cold cereal, consider shredded wheat or all-bran.

● Replace bagels with whole-grain crackers, crisp bread or melba toast.

● Replace the white flour in recipes with whole-wheat flour.

● Sprinkle wheat germ on yogurt and salads for a fiber kick.

● Buy whole-wheat pasta and bread.

● Substitute brown rice for white rice.

● Use fruit as the cornerstone of your snacks. For instance, preheat oven for 350° F. Slice a whole-wheat English muffin in half, top with apple slices and shredded low-fat cheese. Bake just until cheese melts.

● Consider baked apples or peaches as a dessert option. Core the fruit, sprinkle with cinnamon and bake at 350° F for 15 minutes.

Sample Week 9 Eat More Fiber Goals:
This week, I will switch from white bread to whole-grain bread.

or

I will try to eat three whole grains per day and at least three servings of fruits and vegetables.

or

For my coffee break at work, I will eat a piece of fruit.

Your Week 9 Eat More Fiber Goals:

_____

_____

_____

_____

_____

_____

_____

Your Fruit & Vegetables

Use the check-off sheet on these pages to keep
you're eating each day. The goal is to get three

Sunday	Monday	Tuesday
❑	❑	❑
❑	❑	❑
❑	❑	❑
❑	❑	❑
❑	❑	❑
❑	❑	❑
❑	❑	❑
❑	❑	❑
❑	❑	❑
❑	❑	❑
❑	❑	❑
❑	❑	❑
❑	❑	❑
❑	❑	❑
❑	❑	❑
❑	❑	❑
❑	❑	❑
❑	❑	❑
❑	❑	❑
❑	❑	❑

Check-Off List

track of the number of fruits and vegetables
to five servings of these daily.

Wednesday	Thursday	Friday	Saturday
❑	❑	❑	❑
❑	❑	❑	❑
❑	❑	❑	❑
❑	❑	❑	❑
❑	❑	❑	❑
❑	❑	❑	❑
❑	❑	❑	❑
❑	❑	❑	❑
❑	❑	❑	❑
❑	❑	❑	❑
❑	❑	❑	❑
❑	❑	❑	❑
❑	❑	❑	❑
❑	❑	❑	❑
❑	❑	❑	❑
❑	❑	❑	❑
❑	❑	❑	❑
❑	❑	❑	❑
❑	❑	❑	❑
❑	❑	❑	❑

Your Whole Grains

Use this check-off sheet on these pages to
are eating each day. The goal is to get three

Sunday	Monday	Tuesday
☐	☐	☐
☐	☐	☐
☐	☐	☐
☐	☐	☐
☐	☐	☐
☐	☐	☐
☐	☐	☐
☐	☐	☐
☐	☐	☐
☐	☐	☐
☐	☐	☐
☐	☐	☐

Check-Off List

keep track of the number of whole grains you
servings daily of whole-grain products.

Wednesday	Thursday	Friday	Saturday
☐	☐	☐	☐
☐	☐	☐	☐
☐	☐	☐	☐
☐	☐	☐	☐
☐	☐	☐	☐
☐	☐	☐	☐
☐	☐	☐	☐
☐	☐	☐	☐
☐	☐	☐	☐
☐	☐	☐	☐
☐	☐	☐	☐
☐	☐	☐	☐

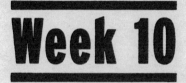

Week 10

Cook Your Own Meals

*I*n our drive-thru culture, there really isn't any reason that you need to learn how to cook — except that you will be healthier if you do. When you are eating in restaurants, you really do not know how your food is prepared or what the portion size is. You also may be getting more hidden sodium than you realize.

For the cost and time of a month of restaurant-eating, you can enroll in a basic cooking class at your local community college, ask mom to help teach you (or maybe that's the reason why you don't know?) or start watching Food TV religiously. The goal here isn't to throw a lavish dinner party, just to be able to feed yourself nutritious fare. In this case, there is another option to "cooking." You can fake it.

The microwave is one of the busiest helpers in your kitchen. It boils, it warms, it makes meals in minutes. And after you survive a day full of exercise, work and relationships, it's the perfect solution to a quick, easy, healthy meal. The following no-fuss, low-mess options are ideal ways to help fuel your body and keep your diet healthy. Organized by food staples, you will find the basic way to cook the food staple and then a recipe or two to make it a meal. I have also provided microwave tips throughout to help you use the microwave better.

➜ **Mindful Microwave Tip: *All microwaves differ in temperature, so cooking times are approximate.***

Food Staple: Egg Whites

Using either prepared egg whites from a carton or whites you've separated by hand, place the desired amount in a microwave-safe bowl. Set the bowl in the microwave with a paper towel over the top. Cook approximately one minute on high, then stir with a fork. Re-cover bowl and cook approximately one-and-a-half minutes more on high.

→ **Mindful Microwave Tip:** *Keep egg whites covered since they're likely to spatter and create a mess in your microwave.*

Huevos Rancheros

1/4 cup canned turkey chili, like Health Valley or Hormel (with or without beans)

2 corn tortillas

4 egg whites, prepared as above

1/4 cup shredded fat-free cheddar cheese

Heat chili in a microwave-safe bowl for two minutes on high; remove and set aside. Place tortillas between two paper towels and heat in microwave 15 seconds on high or until hot. Remove tortillas to a plate or a flat bowl, then top with cooked egg whites, chili and cheese. *Serves 1.*

Per serving: 275 calories, 29 g protein, 30 g carbohydrate, 4 g fat, 4 g fiber.

Basic Breakfast Burrito

You can add ingredients like black beans to increase the protein or leftover rice to boost the carbohydrates, depending on your nutritional needs.

> **1/4 cup Morningstar Farms soy crumbles**
> **1/4 cup chopped romaine lettuce**
> **1/4 cup diced tomato**
> **6 egg whites, prepared as above**
> **10-inch flour tortilla**

Prepare soy crumbles according to package directions. Meanwhile, place lettuce, tomato and egg whites on top of tortilla. Add crumbles and wrap into a burrito. *Serves 1.*

Per serving: 239 calories, 7 g protein, 41 g carbohydrate, 5 g fat, 3 g fiber.

Food Staple: Lean Ground Turkey & Beef

Place ground turkey in a microwave-safe dish. Cook on high for two minutes, then break meat apart with a fork. Continue heating and breaking meat apart until meat is fully cooked, about six minutes per pound.

➜ Mindful Microwave Tip:
Microwaves cook from the inside out. If you want browned meat, sear it in a pan on the stove before cooking it in the microwave.

Turkey Scramble
6 egg whites, prepared as above
5 oz. lean ground turkey, prepared as above
1/4 cup diced tomato
1 Tbsp. parsley flakes or chopped cilantro

In a bowl, top egg whites with turkey, tomato and parsley. *Serves 1.*

Per serving: 282 calories, 42 g protein, 4 g carbohydrate, 9 g fat, 1 g fiber.

Turkey Vegetable Au Gratin

1 1/2 cups water
2 1/2-lb. spaghetti squash (enough to
    make 3 cups)
3 small zucchini, diced
3 cloves garlic, peeled and minced
14.5-oz. can stewed diced tomatoes
3/4 cup shredded low-fat mozzarella
    cheese, divided
10 oz. lean ground turkey, prepared
    as above

Pour water into a microwave-safe 9-by-11-inch baking dish. Cut spaghetti squash in half and place cut side down in dish. Cover loosely with plastic wrap. Microwave on high 15 to 20 minutes. When squash is done, drain water out of dish and scrape squash flesh into dish with a fork. Dispose of squash shells.

Place zucchini, garlic and tomatoes in a microwave-safe bowl, cover with a paper towel and microwave on high for five minutes. Remove from microwave, then stir in 1/4 cup cheese and turkey.

Mix another 1/4 cup cheese into squash in baking dish. Spoon zucchini/turkey mixture over squash and top with remaining 1/4 cup cheese. Microwave five minutes on high. *Serves 6.*

Per serving: 169 calories, 15 g protein, 10 g carbohydrate, 8 g fat, 1 g fiber.

➜ **Mindful Microwave Tip:** *To ensure you get the most cooking power from your microwave, place items in the center of the oven.*

Food Staple: Fish

In a microwave-safe dish, place 1/4 cup water and 8 ounces of your favorite fish (we used salmon or cod for our recipes). Microwave 10 to 15 minutes on high.

Black Beans, Couscous & Poached Salmon

1 cup water

1/2 cup canned black beans

1/2 cup uncooked couscous

8 oz. salmon, prepared as above

Pour water into a microwave-safe bowl and heat for two minutes on high or until water boils. Remove from microwave and mix in couscous. Cover and let sit five minutes. Meanwhile, place beans in a separate microwave-safe bowl, cover with a paper towel and microwave on high for three minutes. Drain beans, then mix with couscous. Spoon beans/couscous mixture onto a plate and place salmon on top. *Serves 1.*

Per serving: 697 calories, 63 g protein, 87 g carbohydrate, 9 g fat, 13 g fiber.

→ **Mindful Microwave Tip:** *Never put metal items like aluminum foil or tin cans into a microwave oven.*

Fish Tacos
4 corn tortillas
8 oz. white fish, like cod (even fish sticks will work; prepare according to package directions), prepared as above
1/4 cup diced tomato
1/2 cup shredded cabbage
1 Tbsp. chopped cilantro
1 Tbsp. salsa verde

On a large plate, lay two tortillas next to

each other so they just overlap on one side; repeat with the remaining tortillas on a separate plate. Divide fish, tomato, cabbage, cilantro and salsa between each pair of tortillas. Fold up into two tacos. *Serves 1.*

Per serving: 440 calories, 48 g protein, 53 g carbohydrate, 4 g fat, 8 g fiber.

Food Staple: Vegetables

Vegetables are a great side dish to any of the previously mentioned bodybuilding staples. Using the microwave makes preparation quick and simple.

Yams & Baked Potatoes

After scrubbing your spud and pricking it several times with a fork, bake it in the microwave for seven to 10 minutes on high.

➜ **Mindful Microwave Tip:** *For a nearly instant meal, fill yams and potatoes with heated chili or steamed vegetables.*

Steamed Vegetables

Place vegetable of choice in a microwave-safe dish with about a half-inch of water at the bottom. Heat five to seven minutes on high or to desired tenderness.

➜ Mindful Microwave Tip: *If you use plastic containers in the microwave, don't secure the top tightly since pressure may build and burst the container. Never re-use old food containers in the microwave; they aren't considered microwave-safe.*

Stock Your Kitchen for Speedy Success

To ensure you're in and out of the kitchen in no time, use this shopping list to make your meals quick and easy.

PRODUCE SECTION

- ❑ Yams
- ❑ Potatoes (new or baking)
- ❑ Carrots
- ❑ Broccoli
- ❑ Squash (spaghetti, acorn or zucchini)
- ❑ Spinach
- ❑ Cabbage
- ❑ Tomatoes
- ❑ Cilantro
- ❑ Lettuce

MEAT SECTION

- ❑ Salmon
- ❑ Cod
- ❑ Ground turkey
- ❑ Ground beef

FREEZER SECTION

- ❑ Soy sausage patties (I like Morningstar Farms brand)
- ❑ Fish sticks (I like Van de Kamp's Crisp & Healthy brand)
- ❑ Chicken pot stickers (I like the specialty grocery store Trader Joe's brand)
- ❑ Soy crumbles (I like Boca Burger brand)

PANTRY

- ❑ Canned stewed, diced tomatoes (plain, Italian-style or roasted garlic)
- ❑ Salsa verde
- ❑ Parsley
- ❑ Corn tortillas
- ❑ Flour tortillas

REFRIGERATOR SECTION

- ❑ Low-fat cheese
- ❑ Eggs or egg whites

Do's and Don'ts

DON'T microwave an egg in its shell; you could have a messy explosion. Don't microwave an egg out of its shell without piercing the yolk to allow venting.

DON'T microwave whole spherical fruits or vegetables (such as apples and potatoes) without piercing the skin to prevent steam buildup.

DON'T re-use plastic food containers, such as margarine tubs, in the microwave. Chemicals can leech out of non-microwave-able plastics into your food.

DON'T use product wrapping unless it's specifically approved for microwave use.

DON'T let plastic wrap touch your food during microwaving. Place microwave-safe plastic wrap loosely over food, says the U.S. Food and Drug Administration. Some labels indicate that you should leave at least one inch of space between the plastic wrap and the food.

DO cover messy foods like chili, spaghetti sauce and soup to prevent splattering.

DON'T use patterned or colored paper towels and napkins in the microwave. They tend to bleed their designs onto the food or the floor of your microwave. Use only white towels for a clean and easy zap.

DO be aware of the cooking time specified for your microwave recipe. Most are written to accommodate a standard 700-watt appliance. If yours is significantly more powerful, decrease the cooking time accordingly.

DON'T leave plastic lids on tight. Open the vents if lids have them or loosen lids to allow steam to escape.

DO handle hot dishes carefully when removing from the microwave. And be careful when removing lids or coverings or opening bags.

DON'T use metal in the microwave. You already know this, but we just wanted to offer a reminder to be safe.

DO read and follow directions in the owner's manual for your microwave, as well as those on food products and cookware packages.

Sample Week 10 Cook Your Own Meals Goals:

This week, I will sign up for a cooking class.

or

At least three times this week, I will pack my lunch.

or

I will make dinner three times this week (and that doesn't mean calling for takeout).

Your Week 10 Cook Your Own Meals Goals:

_____

_____

_____

_____

_____

_____

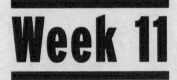

Stocking Up

During this time when you are trying to abandon fast-food restaurants and forge a healthy way of living, it is frustrating to have passed up the convenience of drive-thru restaurants only to stand in front of the refrigerator or pantry to find nothing to eat. Your stomach is growling — it's enough to make you downright cranky. So much for a relaxing evening at home.

Instead of calling your neighborhood Domino's, this chapter will prepare you to have emergency rations on hand so you can make good-for-you meals on the fly. I live by having these easy-to-store and even easier-to-prepare staples on hand. It allows me to not think about meal planning when the last thing that I want to do is think.

Packing the Pantry

Keeping a well-stocked pantry will help you avoid the takeout trap. The key is to purchase such items as low- or no-sodium canned goods. Look for items where the milligrams of sodium are equal to or less than the calories. Here is what you should have on hand:

Fruits & Vegetables
❑ Canned diced tomatoes with Italian herbs
❑ Spaghetti sauce
❑ Pizza sauce
❑ Salsa
❑ Diced tomatoes with green chiles
❑ Artichoke hearts
❑ Baby corn
❑ Roasted bell peppers
❑ Julienned carrot sticks
❑ Canned fruit, like pineapple, mandarin oranges, peaches, etc.
❑ Dried fruit

Grains & Starches
❑ Boil-in-the-bag rice, brown is preferred but white is OK, too.

❑ Pasta, any variety
❑ High-fiber cereal (3 or more grams of fiber per serving)
❑ Bread crumbs
❑ Whole-grain crackers

Proteins

❑ Canned tuna, salmon, chicken, clams, crabmeat
❑ Variety of canned beans
❑ Nuts and seeds

Oils & Such

❑ Olive oil
❑ Canola oil
❑ Peanut oil
❑ Sesame oil
❑ Chili oil
❑ Red wine vinegar
❑ White wine vinegar
❑ Rice vinegar
❑ Balsamic vinegar
❑ Light salad dressings
❑ Stir-fry or teriyaki sauce

The Well-Stocked Refrigerator

I have an aunt whose refrigerator is busting with stuff. You can't find anything in it. And you definitely can't find something to make. The moral is that a well-stocked refrigerator doesn't necessarily mean it is full. To be able to whip up healthy foods, here is what you should have:

❑ Eggs
❑ Fat-free milk
❑ Low-fat cheeses
❑ Fat-free plain yogurt
❑ Wheat germ
❑ Whole-grain bread (2 grams of fiber per slice is optimal)
❑ Long-lasting vegetables, like onions, celery, carrots and bell peppers
❑ Light mayonnaise
❑ Light salad dressing
❑ Mustard
❑ Lemon and lime juices
❑ Light soy sauce

Freezer Rations

The freezer is a great place to have your emergency rations, as food still tastes fresh once cooked. And the best thing is that frozen foods are getting more sophisticated. You can now buy precooked poultry that is low in sodium and preservatives. Grocery stores are now offering marinated meats that can be used for stir-fry or fajitas. There are also meals in the bag that can offer a host of possibilities. Again, you'll want to watch the sodium. Stock your freezer with these essentials:

Fruits & Vegetables
- Stir-fry mixes
- Chopped onions and/or peppers
- Broccoli florets
- Carrots
- Asparagus spears
- Corn
- Chopped spinach
- Baby brussels sprouts
- Peaches
- Blueberries
- Strawberries
- Mixed berries

Grains and Complex Carbs

- ❑ Pizza crust
- ❑ Bagels
- ❑ Tortillas
- ❑ Fresh pasta

Protein

- ❑ Thinly sliced or cubed sirloin steak
- ❑ Lean ground meat
- ❑ Skinless chicken tenders
- ❑ Egg substitute
- ❑ Soy sausage
- ❑ Fully cooked chicken breast
- ❑ Cooked shrimp
- ❑ Fish fillets

Snack Suggestions

You never know when hunger may strike. So it is important that you keep food on hand that is easy to prepare and satisfies any cravings you may have. Use this list as a guide for emergency snacking rations:

- ❑ Almond, cashew or peanut butters
- ❑ Whole-grain bagels

❑ Low-fat microwave popcorn
❑ Pretzels
❑ Fig bars
❑ Fudgsicles
❑ Ginger snaps
❑ Frozen yogurt
❑ Sorbet
❑ Sports bars and drinks
❑ Fruit juice
❑ Dried fruits and nuts
❑ Trail mix

Your New Cooking Staples

Below are cooking suggestions using the above ingredients.

Breakfast Ideas

● High-fiber cereal and milk
● Regular-flavored oatmeal mixed with applesauce
● One cup plain yogurt mixed with thawed berries, topped with wheat germ
● Scrambled eggs and soy sausage

- Breakfast burrito: scrambled eggs and cheese wrapped in a tortilla, topped with salsa
- Omelet made with eggs, bell peppers, black beans, cheese and salsa
- Omelet made with broccoli florets and cheese
- Toasted bagel with peanut butter and a glass of juice
- Smoothie made from your choice of frozen fruit blended with nonfat milk and wheat germ

Lunch or Dinner Ideas

- Mix a can of white or black beans with a can of tuna or salmon. Add celery, red onions and a little red wine vinegar, olive oil and cumin.
- Make your own pizza with a frozen pizza shell, cheese, pizza sauce and top with frozen vegetables.
- Flavor fish fillets with lemon juice and bread crumbs. Cook in the microwave four to six minutes. Serve with your favorite vegetable and quick-cooking rice.
- Brown chicken tenders in skillet for 10

minutes. Transfer to baking dish and cover with salsa and shredded cheese. Bake for 10 minutes at 400 degrees F. Serve with quick-cooking rice.

● Stir-fry vegetables with cooked shrimp and serve over rice.

● Make fish tacos. Bake frozen fish fillets per package instructions. Serve in corn tortillas with shredded cabbage and salsa.

● Mix canned tuna or salmon with 1 Tbsp. of light mayonnaise and chopped celery. Serve between two slices of whole-grain bread. Pair with an apple or glass of milk.

● Mix cooked pasta with either cooked shrimp or cooked chicken breast. Top with spaghetti sauce. Serve with a small salad.

● Using bagged lettuce, create your own salad. A suggestion is using bagged spinach, toss with dried apricots, chopped walnuts and goat cheese and use balsamic vinegar for the dressing. Or mix together black beans, tomatoes, avocado, cooked chicken or shrimp and top with fat-free sour cream for a taco salad.

● Fajitas. Pan-sear pre-marinated meat and mix with bell peppers and onions. Serve with tortillas and salsa.

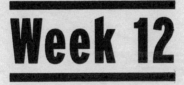

Week 12

Dairy

*T*o lose weight, you have to drink milk. If you are like many who have ditched the dairy to maintain your waistline, you should know that scientific research has found that eating high amounts of calcium-rich dairy products in general, and specifically milk, yogurt and cheese, actually correlates to weight loss.

Milk-drinkers weigh less and enjoy a lower percentage of body fat than milk-avoiders. Research has found that dieters who follow dairy-rich meal plans lose more weight, and more fat, than do those who shun dairy altogether. Long-term data tell us that people who eat large amounts of calcium in the form of dairy are leaner and lighter than those who avoid dairy.

Why is this? There is a little-known hormone in our body called calcitriol. When your body doesn't get enough calcium, it produces calcitriol to preserve calcium. While preserving the calcium in your system, calcitriol also stimulates the production and the storage of fat and reduces fat breakdown. Dietary calcium can prevent and reverse this process, triggering "fat-burning" hormones to break down and release fat while suppressing the formation of new fat.

In fact, dietary calcium can also enhance thermogenesis (the process of your body creating heat), allowing your cells to burn more calories, helping you burn fat and lose weight. Bottom line: A low-calcium diet causes your fat cells to get even bigger. Dietary calcium helps them shrink.

Among the most promising findings from dairy research is that the women who followed weight-loss diets high in calcium-rich foods were able to preserve and sometimes gain lean body mass, thereby increasing their metabolic rate over time. (Experts say that for every pound of muscle your body burns 30 to 50 calories each day.)

In spring 2002, General Mills sponsored

a study in which subjects were randomly assigned to one of two diet groups. Both diets prescribed 500 fewer calories per day than the subjects were eating before the intervention. One meal plan included three 6-ounce servings of Yoplait light yogurt; the other called for three servings of sugar-free Jell-o (and no supplemental calcium).

While both groups lost weight, probably from the 500-calorie deficit, the yogurt-eaters lost 22 percent more weight, 61 percent more body fat and 81 percent more abdominal fat than their Jell-O-eating counterparts. The yogurt-eaters also maintained more lean body mass than their peers — about twice as much.

What's most surprising, though, is that on average they lost more than an inch in waist circumference during the study, a loss six times greater than the non-yogurt eaters.

Boning Up

Another important health boost from a high-calcium diet relates to bone density. Too many Americans suffer from the brittle-bone disease osteoporosis. Unfortunately, even modest weight loss can further compromise bone density. By keeping the calcium level up while cutting calories, you may be able to sidestep this negative effect. Eating more dairy products provides enough calcium to exceed the common recommendations for bone health (approximately 1,000 milligrams a day) and may help minimize the bone loss often associated with calorie restriction and weight loss.

Will Supplementation Work?

You've got so much on your plate right now and adding dairy to your diet might just be more than you can chew. So, you're wondering: Can you take a shortcut and take a calcium supplement instead? The answer: Not really.

One study that compared supplemental calcium, dairy calcium and low-calcium diets found that people eating dairy still lost the most weight of the three groups. Though women who used supplemental calcium were better off than those consuming diets lacking both dairy and supplements, their weight loss didn't match that of the women following dairy-rich diets. Numerous weight-loss studies confirm that as calcium intake goes up, body weight and body fat go down.

Researchers believe that, like the polyphenols in wine and the phytochemicals in leafy greens, dairy products contain a host of biologically active compounds — nutrients that work synergistically with the calcium to assist with weight loss and weight regulation. Calcium supplements just can't mimic the properties of the real thing.

Bloated Matters

Does milk sour or upset your stomach? Lactose intolerance can make getting enough calcium a challenge. This condition is characterized by an inability to digest lactose — a milk sugar found in dairy products — which leads to intestinal gas and bloating. A study out of the University of Tennessee focused exclusively on African-Americans, a group thought to be susceptible to lactose intolerance. Only two of the 36 participants reported complications of lactose intolerance, which is easily remedied by taking over-the-counter lactase enzymes that digest milk sugar. The participants also tolerated aged cheeses and fermented dairy products quite well (these foods are generally better tolerated by lactose-intolerant people).

While those with more aggressive symptoms unfortunately need to rely on the use of enzyme tablets to ease digestion, there are so many options available today — from treated milk to treated ice cream — that lactose-free dairy products should be easy to find and incorporate into your diet.

If dairy does a number on you, try slowly building up the amount of dairy you consume over time; keep the serving sizes small; consume dairy products with meals; choose aged cheeses with less lactose, and drink lactose-free milk. For more information on lactose intolerance, check out: the National Digestive Diseases Information Clearinghouse at www.niddk.nih.gov/health/digest/pubs/lactose/lactose.htm and the U.S. National Library of Medicine at www.nlm.nih.gov/medlineplus/ency/article/000276.htm.

If you just don't like dairy, getting enough calcium without supplementation can be a challenge. While it's true that there are a variety of other foods that are rich in calcium, dairy is still the best bet. The research that connects calcium to weight loss so far has been done with dairy products. Many green vegetables contain calcium; the problem is that these foods also contain phytates, compounds that bind with calcium and prevent its absorption. You'd need to eat more than eight cups of broccoli to match the amount of calcium in three cups of milk and most of the calcium in the broccoli wouldn't be absorbed.

If you are a vegan, calcium-fortified soymilk will meet your needs fairly well. Fortified soymilk contains a well-absorbed form of calcium that's equivalent to a good calcium supplement, if not better. However, there is no evidence to determine whether calcium-fortified soy will produce the same results as dairy on weight loss.

How Much Is Enough?

While four servings of dairy per day would be optimal — yet may be difficult to do — three servings are a must. Choose low-fat or fat-free milk and yogurt and experiment with reduced-fat cheeses. While cheese is a great source of protein and calcium, it is also higher in saturated fat. Instead, focus on the addition of milk and yogurt to make up your high-dairy diet. That way, you'll get the same amount of protein and calcium without all the saturated fat and additional calories.

A serving of dairy should contain approximately 300 mg of calcium. One cup of milk, one cup (8 ounces) of yogurt or 1.5 ounces of cheese all contain approximately 300 mg of calcium. Eating a minimum of three servings of dairy provides 900 mg of calcium. Since the average American diet provides between 500 and 600 mg of non-dairy calcium, your goal is to get about 1,200 mg — 1,500 mg of calcium.

You may not want to drink three glasses of milk every day. For more variety, mix it up. Stock up on low-fat/fat-free yogurt for breakfast, midday snacks or a guilt-free dessert. Combine milk and yogurt into a fruit smoothie. Add cheese to your sandwiches and experiment with healthy lasagna. (I've given you an easy recipe on the next page.)

Ray's Fool-Proof Lasagna

1 package frozen chopped spinach
1 package (16 oz.) lasagna noodles
1 quart (32 oz.) Ragu Plain Spaghetti Sauce
1 lb. fresh Italian sausage, mild (use any variety)
1 package sliced low-fat mozzarella cheese
1 package shredded low-fat mozzarella cheese
Garlic powder to taste
Oregano and parmesan cheese to taste

Preheat oven to 350° F. Cook noodles and drain as directed. Fry sausage without casing and season with garlic powder. Drain off fat, add spaghetti sauce and simmer approximately 45 minutes. Cook spinach according to package directions and drain very well.

Assembly: Pour 1/4 cup sauce on the bottom of the pan and then layer the pan with noodles. Next place the spinach and the cheese. Continue layering sauce, noodles, spinach, cheese. Top with slices of mozzarella cheese. Sprinkle with oregano and parmesan. Bake loosely covered with aluminum foil for 25 minutes. *Serves 12.*

Nondairy Sources of Calcium

Food	Amount	Calcium (mg)
Tofu	1/2 cup	260
Soy milk	1 cup	varies
Almonds	1 oz.	80
Sardines	3 oz.	180
Sesame seeds, toasted	1 oz.	280
Navy beans	1 cup cooked	125
White beans	1 cup cooked	160
Broccoli (frozen)	1 cup cooked	94
Kale	1 cup cooked	95
Mustard greens	1 cup cooked	100
Chinese cabbage (bok choy)	1 cup cooked	160
Turnip greens	1 cup cooked	200
Spinach	1 cup cooked	245

Milk Products

Product	Calories	Protein	Carbs	Fat
Measurement: 1 cup		(g)	(g)	(g)
Nonfat milk	80	9	12	0
Low-fat milk (1% fat)	100	8	11	3
Reduced-fat milk (2% fat)	120	8	11	5
Whole milk	150	8	11	8
Chocolate milk, low-fat	90	8	11	1
Lactose-free, fat-free (Lactaid)	80	8	13	0
Buttermilk, low-fat (1% fat)	100	9	12	2.5
Goat's milk	140	8	11	7
Soy milk, fat-free, plain	80	3	15	0
Soy milk plus	140	6	19	4
Soy milk, chocolate, low-fat	140	6	23	3

Sample Week 12 Dairy Goals:

I will drink a glass of skim milk before each meal.

or

I will snack on yogurt at least three times this week.

or

I will cook the yummy lasagna recipe that is in this chapter.

Your Week 12 Dairy Goals:

_____

_____

_____

_____

_____

_____

_____

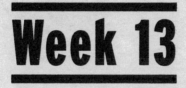

Sweetening of America

*T*he white, refined granulates keep beckoning the taste buds of America. Whether in the form of sugar or as high-fructose corn syrup, there is such a range of non-sugar products today that for our purposes here we will call them caloric sweeteners. In the United States, between 1977 and 1996, there was a remarkable increase of 83 calories of caloric sweetener consumed per day by everyone ages 2 and older. The percentage of the American diet consisting of caloric sweeteners rose from 13.1 to 16 percent and between the years 1994 and 1996, more than 30 percent of the carbohydrates that we consumed came from caloric sweeteners.

Why do we have such a taste for the sweet stuff? Keith Ayoob, EdD, RD, associate professor at Albert Einstein College of Medicine in New York City told *Muscle & Fitness Hers*: "It's something that's in us. Most people have a preference for sweetness. When sugar consumption is out of control, it's due to environment, availability or both. Relatively speaking, it's a pretty cheap experience. A quick fix, but not long-lasting. People end up feeling guilty."

Think about it. Do you reach into your co-worker's candy dish when the two of you are just gabbing? Or do you seek it out when the going starts getting tough? As children, candy might have been a reward to you. As an adult, something sweet may still be your reward. My friend Natasha picks up a pint of ice cream after a particularly grueling day at work because in her mind she deserves it.

The thing is: Sugar isn't necessarily bad for you, but too much of the sweet stuff can cause havoc, such as if you make a pronounced shift in your diet toward increased consumption of caloric sweeteners and away from high-fiber foods that provide energy in the form of calories but few other nutrients.

The purpose of this book is to promote better eating habits and better food choices; therefore, we're not going to attempt to eliminate sugar and other caloric sweeteners from your diet. We are going to try and reduce the amount that you eat. This makes it easier to adopt a long-lasting behavior and attitude toward sugar. Therefore, we will not try to prescribe a set amount of caloric sweeteners for you to eat — it would be too difficult. Instead, we are attacking this caloric taboo in other ways — such as drinking more non-caloric drinks like water since most caloric drinks are sweetened with high-fructose corn syrup.

Can You Be Addicted to Sugar?

Addiction requires three elements: increased intake and changes in brain chemistry; upon deprivation, signs of withdrawal and further changes in brain chemistry, and craving and relapse after withdrawal is over.

Unlike a drug-addicted junkie, you probably won't be robbing a convenience store in the near future to support your sugar habit. But when you're hungry, you probably seek the quick fix that sugary carbohydrates provide. Never fear, for all addictions there is rehab. In the refrigerator of life, there is behavior modification.

First, figure out what triggers you to reach for those sweet treats. Look at your food diary and ask yourself the following questions:

- *What is happening to you before you binge?*
- *What time of the day/week/month do you indulge in your sweet craving?*
- *What are you eating before the sweet stuff? Does it make you crave the sweet stuff?*
- *Are you hungry or what is your level of hunger when you crave sweets?*

After doing this troubleshooting, you may find that some of these factors might be uncontrollable. At that point, it is time to make sweets less available. To do this:

- *Ask co-workers to keep the goodies in their offices.*

• *Keep a bowl of fruit at your desk to satisfy sweet cravings.*

• *Ask your spouse not to bring home candy or other sugar-laden foods.*

• *If you have been buying the big candy bar, opt for the smaller size.*

The Sweetest Success

Learning how to moderate caloric sweeteners and manage their consumption can help you adopt a diet that will help you lose weight and help you ward off disease. People tend to binge on sugar when they have been avoiding it for long periods of time. Our goal here will be to incorporate sugar into your diet so that it only is 10 percent of your total daily caloric intake, or about 100 to 200 calories per day. Here are some tips to keep your daily treat within your needs:

• **Make sure you don't skip meals.** This may make you reach for sugar-laden treats.

• **Treat yourself occasionally**, even daily, using the suggestions below.

• **Don't sliver.** A sliver of cake, a bite of a cookie, a piece of candy and similar small mouthfuls can add up throughout the day.

Instead, make your sweet treat a reasonable size, large enough to satisfy you but small enough that you don't throw off your nutritional balance.

• **Have one truffle**, eaten slowly and savored.

• **Dip fresh fruit** in chocolate or caramel sauce (about 2 tablespoons of syrup).

• **Dried fruits.** Think beyond raisins; try apricot, mango, papaya and dates. A quarter-cup is about 100 calories.

• **One-half of a restaurant dessert** (or less). Make it a personal philosophy that desserts are meant to be shared.

Sample Week 13 Sweetening of America Goals:

This week, I will have a piece of fruit instead of a candy bar for a snack.

or

This week, I will have only one full-calorie soda per day.

or

For my coffee break at work, I will go for a 10-minute walk instead of walking to the vending machine.

Your Week 13 Sweetening of America Goals:

_____

_____

_____

_____

_____

_____

_____

_____

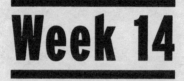

Week 14

Exercise

Want a fun way to get stronger, leaner and feel more energetic all day long? It's an answer you've heard before: Start an exercise program.

Now, before you dismiss it — maybe you think you just don't have time or perhaps you just feel intimidated walking into a health club — read this chapter. Perhaps by the end, we'll find a way to make all your reservations about starting a fitness program disappear. It's certainly not as difficult or time-consuming as most people think, I promise you!

Of course, unless you've been living under a rock, you know that exercising on a regular basis is a good idea. Science has proven beyond a shadow of a doubt that those who exercise dramatically improve their health, their quality of life and their life span. Here are some of the more notable facts of what exercise can do for you:

✔ **Improves your heart health and fights off cardiovascular disease.** As the sedentary nature of modern-day life takes its toll on our waistlines and fast food slowly clogs our arteries, heart disease has skyrocketed to epidemic proportions. But there is hope and it doesn't require you to run 20 miles a day and never eat a french fry again. A moderate bout of daily exercise, as little as a 30-minute brisk walk per day, can greatly reduce your risk factors for heart disease.

✔ **Makes you stronger.** Tired of feeling wiped out after carrying in the groceries? Don't let general muscle weakness limit your daily activities. Sure, when you're in your 20s and early 30s it's not so noticeable, but as you get older, muscle atrophy can take a huge toll on your quality of life. But as little as 20 minutes of resistance training three times per week can make a noticeable improvement in your strength levels. You may not be competing in a strongman contest anytime soon, but you will be able to stay active well into your later years. It's a wise investment, one that you won't regret while you're on the golf course at age 70!

✔ **Helps you look better.** Toned, shapely muscles and less body fat are the most well-known byproduct of a fitness regimen. Who wants to be the tub o' lard at the neighborhood pool party? With a little exercise, you can build a body that you can be proud of — wouldn't it be nice to never have to hide under a T-shirt at the beach again?

✔ **Releases your stress.** This is a benefit you may not automatically associate with exercise, but it's a proven fact — exercise helps you relieve feelings of stress and anxiety. Physical activity causes the body to release endorphins, which improve your mood and help you beat the blues.

✔ **Increases your brainpower.** Training helps you develop a synergy between your mind and body. After a few weeks, you'll soon discover you're more alert, aware and ready to take on any challenges that arise.

✔ **Amps up your energy levels.** Being sluggish is a common problem in our society, with lots of time spent at work, and money and family pressures draining us physically and emotionally. With brief bouts of exercise, you can battle back, priming your body to be an efficient user and producer of energy.

✔ **Strengthens your bones.** Exercise is often associated with building muscle, but it increases your bone density, as well. Along with a solid nutritional strategy, regular training with weights is a proven way to help prevent a common ailment in older adults: osteoporosis. Strong, healthy bones can keep you vital today and in the future.

✔ **Delays aging.** We're all looking for that fountain of youth. People seek it in creams, potions and even plastic surgery in the most extreme cases. The Fountain of Youth may not exist in a physical sense — there's no body of water on Earth that'll turn back the hands of time — but there is something that can slow the aging process. Yes, you guessed it, it's exercise.

Science has shown that it slows common markers of aging. Make fitness a part of your life and you can look younger for much longer.

✔ **Teaches you self-control.** So much of what goes wrong with our bodies and in our lives is truly under our control. We choose what we eat, we choose whether we live a sedentary or an active lifestyle, we decide whether we want to take life by the horns and live it to its fullest or whether we sit back and let situations and circumstances beat down our spirit.

Choosing to exercise, and then sticking with it until it becomes a habit, is a decision that will spill over into every area of your life. Willpower is a trait that can be learned and can be strengthened over time with use, just like a muscle. Through fitness you learn discipline and you begin to take control over your own body and health. It is an exhilarating process — you'll find that once you reach a certain point, you're hooked.

Millions of people have made exercise a regular part of their life and, indeed, look forward to that part of their day. That can be you, too, if you give it time and stick with it. Talk to people who do it and you'll find they remember "turning a corner," when exercise transformed from being something they worked at to something they enjoyed and would never want to give up. Hang in there and it will happen!

✔ **Helps alleviate any need to crash diet.** While you can't use exercise as an excuse to eat anything you want, it does help provide you some leeway in what you eat. You don't have to watch every single morsel of food you take in if you're taking the initiative to stay active.

Exercise boosts your body's metabolism naturally — over time, your body will burn more calories, even at rest. Thus, you can better balance the calories coming in with calories being expended and that is truly the key for maintaining a healthy weight.

Take a Dip Into the Fitness Water

So you're sold — you'd like to take the next step and dip your toe into the waters of fitness. You certainly don't have to go overboard, as I mentioned early on in this chapter. No endless hours of running or lifting — in fact, the last thing you should do at this point is go full-bore into a program. So many people jump with both feet into an exercise program, trying hard to work out five or six days a week, only to burn themselves out to the point where they dread ever going back into a gym. It's the New Year's resolution phenomenon — hundreds of thousands of people flock to health clubs in January every year, plunk down their money for a membership, work out religiously for a few weeks, then give up as suddenly as they began, disenchanted (and very, very sore!).

You should play it smart. Start easy and slow — at the beginning, you should stop exercising well before you feel like you've really done anything. For instance, you could start walking around your neighborhood for 20 minutes, three days per week. On your first few forays out, you may get to 20 minutes and say, "I feel good — I'm going to keep going!" When that happens, though, don't do it! Stick to your time limits. While this example is not directly comparable, it is related; seasoned athletes often talk about "leaving something on the practice field," stopping before they are completely drained of energy. It's a good lesson — if you stop exercising while you still feel like you can do more, you give yourself impetus to return. You have more to give for next time. You come in to each session rarin' to go, instead of still sore and weak from your previous workout.

With that said, here are some sample programs you can use, just to get you started in fitness. Use these for one to three months. After that time, you'll be ready and hopefully more than willing to step up your efforts a bit. At that point, you could consult a personal trainer who can put you on a slightly more challenging program or consult a fitness book from a certified professional. Magazines such as *Muscle & Fitness* (or *Muscle & Fitness Hers*) can also provide valuable information for exercisers of all levels.

Program 1: At-Home

You'll walk for your cardiovascular workout and perform simple exercises that can be done in the comfort of your own home for the resistance portion of your training.

Perform the following on three nonconsecutive days each week, such as a Monday, Wednesday and Friday. In total, it should only take 45 minutes maximum.

CARDIO:

Brisk walk (outdoors or on a treadmill, if you have one): 20 minutes.

RESISTANCE:

Body weight Squat (three sets of 10 repetitions): Stand with your feet shoulder-width apart, hands on your hips or on your shoulders. With your chest puffed out, head up and back slightly arched, bend your knees and shift your hips back as if you were going to sit back in a chair. Stop when your thighs reach a position parallel to the floor, then reverse the motion by straightening your knees and shifting your hips forward. On the ascent, you can better engage your legs by thinking about pressing through your heels to lift yourself up. Once down and up is a "repetition."

Push-Up (three sets of 10 repetitions): This is just like the military-type variety we all know and love. Get face-down on the floor, your hands spaced about shoulder-width apart, your lower body balanced over your toes (if this is too hard, you can start by keeping your knees on the floor until you get stronger). From an arms extended position, and keeping your body straight and flat as a board the entire time, bend your elbows and lower your body until your chest is about an inch from the floor, then reverse to the beginning.

Milk-Jug Row (three sets of 10 repetitions): For these, you'll need two gallon jugs of milk — you can also use jugs that are emptied of milk and have water in them. Stand with your knees slightly bent and bend over from the hips, maintaining the natural arch in your back and keeping your chin up. Grasp the handle of a jug in each hand and hold them with your arms straight and toward the floor. Simultaneously bend your elbows and lift the jugs to each side of your torso — at the top your elbows should be fully bent and pointed at the ceiling — then reverse the motion until your arms are straight again. Repeat for 10 repetitions. If you find the jugs are too heavy when completely full, dump an even amount of milk or water out of each one until the weight is light enough for you to get 10 repetitions relatively easily.

Crunch (three sets of 10 repetitions): Lie face up on the floor with your feet either up in the air or flat on the floor, knees bent. Cross your arms over your chest or place them lightly behind your head. Curl your torso up by contracting your abdominal muscles, simultaneously pressing your lower back into the floor. This is a very small movement, only a few inches, but if you're doing it correctly you should feel the muscles in your midsection (stomach area) tense strongly. Lower yourself back to the floor for a brief second and repeat for 10 reps. As you tire, avoid the tendency to pull on your head with your hands if you are using the hands-behind-your-head position.

Rest one minute between each set.

Program 2: Health Club

For those who want to join a local health club, this resistance machine-based program will help you ease into working out. (Make sure to join one within 20 minutes of your house, as it's been shown that joining a place farther than that makes you more likely to drop out.) If you're unsure about a piece of equipment listed here, ask one of the staff at the gym to direct you. Perform this workout on three nonconsecutive days each week; it should take about 45 minutes total.

RESISTANCE:

Machine Leg Press (two sets of 12 repetitions): Sit comfortably on the horizontal seat so your shoulders fit snugly under the pads and your feet are shoulder-width or slightly wider apart on the upper two-thirds of the foot platform. Pressing through your heels, press until your knees are straight (but not locked), then lower yourself back to a knees-bent position. Don't let the weight stack touch down between repetitions, as that allows your muscles to rest and makes the exercise a bit less effective overall.

Machine Row (two sets of 12 repetitions): This machine works your back muscles. Sit in the seat so that your chest is pressed firmly against the pad and your feet are set solidly on the floor. Take a palms-down or a palms-facing-each-other grip on the handles, then pull evenly to bring your elbows back behind your body. Once you pull the handles back as far as you can, pause and return to the start, again not letting the weight stack touch down before continuing on to the next rep.

Seated Shoulder Machine Press (two sets of 12 repetitions): Sit on the bench so that when you grab the handles, your elbows are directly underneath your hands. The seat should be set so the handles are at shoulder level in the bottom position. Press the handles upward, extending your arms until your elbows are almost straight — don't lock them out — then return to an arms-bent position.

Pec-Deck Flye Machine (two sets of 12 repetitions): Sit squarely on a pec-deck machine, which works your chest (pectoral) muscles. Your back should be pressed into the back of the seat and your forearms and elbows should be on the corresponding pads with your hands grasping the handles. Evenly bring the handles in front of you until they touch directly in front of the center of your chest, then return to a position where the pads are straight out to each side.

Vertical Biceps Curl Machine (one set of 15 repetitions): Adjust the seat so that your upper arms and elbows rest comfortably on the pad, armpits tucked into the edge. Take a shoulder-width grip on the handles and, keeping your elbows in line with your hands, curl the handles toward your shoulders until your arms are fully bent. Pause for a moment at the top, then lower to the start, stopping just short of allowing the weight stack to touch down before beginning the next rep.

Triceps Cable Pressdown (one set of 15 repetitions): Stand upright and grasp a short, straight bar attached to a high cable pulley. It helps if you choose a bar that has a "rotating sleeve" — in this type of cable attachment, the straight shaft of the bar is allowed to rotate within the handle; thus, making it more comfortable as you do this exercise. Keeping your upper arms locked at your sides (the only part of your body that should move is your forearms), press the bar down until your elbows are extended. Return the bar up to a point where your forearms are parallel to the floor and repeat. On this exercise, make sure your body stays upright — leaning forward allows your shoulders to take on the work instead of the intended target, your triceps muscles on the back of your arms.

Decline Crunch (two sets of 15 repetitions): Lie back on a decline bench set to about a 45-degree angle. Cross your arms over your chest or place your hands lightly behind your head. Curl your torso up off of the bench, closing the distance between your pelvis and your rib cage (your abdominal muscles should strongly flex), then lie back to the starting position. To make the move more challenging, try not to let your back curl all the way back down to the bench between each rep — stop an inch or two short and then curl up to the top position.

CARDIO:
Elliptical Trainer or Recumbent Bike: 20 minutes at a comfortable pace.

Sample Week 14 Exercise Goals:

I will walk around the neighborhood for 20 minutes, three days per week.

or

I will do some sort of resistance training three times a week.

or

For my coffee break at work, I will go for a 10-minute walk.

Your Week 14 Exercise Goals:

_____

_____

_____

_____

_____

_____

_____

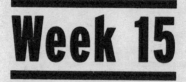

Week 15

Eating Out

Americans work more than ever — more hours per day and even more jobs. More women are in the workplace and about 75 percent of all mothers are in the workforce. No longer do we have time to prepare meals. This is reflected in our love affair with restaurants. In 1993, 38 percent of total food dollars were spent at restaurants. That number increased to 42 percent in 2001 and there is no indication that it is decreasing anytime soon. Researchers Shanthy A. Bowman, Ph.D., and Bryan T. Vineyard, Ph.D., of the Beltsville Human Nutrition Research Center, the Biometrical Consulting Service and the U.S. Department of Agriculture concluded in their study of the effect of fast food on diets:

"As more mothers and meal preparers continue to enter the labor force, they are left with less time for food shopping and food preparation." But this growing fast-food habit may have disastrous effects on our diets.

During their research, which was published in the *Journal of the American College of Nutrition*, Bowman and Vineyard studied the effects of fast food on diet and weight in America. After surveying 9,500 male and female adults, they found that fast-food consumption decreased as age increased. Young adults between the ages of 20 and 29 were four times more likely than adults ages 55 or older to eat at fast-food restaurants.

Those who reported eating fast food had substantially higher calorie, total fat, saturated fat, carbohydrate, added sugars and protein intakes than their nonfast-food-eating counterparts. Fast-food eaters, males and females, had lower intakes of nutritious foods, such as fruits and milk (in its fluid form), than abstainers. They also drank about twice the amount of nondiet carbonated soft drinks than nonfast-food eaters.

When it came to fast food's contribution

to the actual daily caloric intake, fast food made up one-third of the day's calories, total fat and saturated fat. Overall, the fast-food participants' diets were lower in vitamins A and C — two antioxidants that help ward off disease — and the minerals calcium and magnesium, which are associated with bone health. The more often participants ate at fast-food restaurants, the more their calorie and macronutrients increased and micronutrients decreased.

Now for the million-dollar question: Is fast food linked to obesity? If you saw the documentary *Super Size Me?*, you would know that there is some possibility. This study found a small, but significant difference between the mean body mass index values of fast-food eaters and fast-food abstainers. Fast-food eaters had slightly higher and significant odds of being overweight; though Bowman and Vineyard concluded that they could not find a cause-and-effect relationship between fast-food eating and weight gain.

Fast food is so interwoven into the fabric of our society that if you choose to eat it, recognize that it is calorie-dense and choose your food accordingly. A good rule is the smaller the better — a regular hamburger, small chicken nuggets or a taco. With fast- food restaurants like McDonald's and Wendy's adding healthier choices to their menus, food choices may be easier. Check the nutritional postings for these new salads and other "healthy" choices on these restaurants' Web sites to understand their impact on your diet.

The Restaurant Challenge

When we eat away from home, we are offered a large variety of low-cost, energy-dense foods in large portions — all things that encourage us to overeat. The greatest challenge for many is eating at restaurants, where the portions are big and the atmosphere encourages eating for social rather than physical reasons. If you eat out frequently, losing weight and maintaining a healthy weight may be more difficult for you than for someone who eats many meals at home.

A recent study out of the Pennsylvania State University's department of nutrition in the school of hotel, restaurant and recreation management found that in a restaurant setting, increasing the size of an entrée results in increased calorie consumption; supporting the suggestion that large restaurant portions may be contributing to the obesity epidemic.

Once a special treat, restaurants have woven themselves into the framework of our society. No longer are they places to celebrate special occasions. Instead, they have helped develop the structure of our cities as mentioned in the book *Fat Food Nation* and have shaped our palate and resized our waistlines. For us to be truly successful at eating healthy, there are two thoughts about restaurant eating that we need to dismiss: not getting our money's worth and not wasting food.

Some people clean their plates at restaurants because they do not want to waste money or waste food. Ultimately it goes to "waist", the question is which one? And is it really worth the price in health for it to go to "waist"? The excess food is still not feeding your body properly or going to the starving children of the world who need it.

But if restaurant eating is a part of your life,

it is best to come up with a game plan so that all your healthy efforts are not blown by a simple restaurant meal. The nice thing is that restaurants are realizing that their portion sizes may be contributing to the expanding of the American waistline so some chains have taken steps to make it better.

Restaurant Research

The best plans of action are based on intelligence. Most restaurants have Web sites that list the nutritional information of the foods that they serve. By looking up that information, you will be able to prepare your order ahead of time. This way you are thinking about what you'll order, how much you'll eat and whether you can split a dish with someone else. Or vow to ask your server to pack half your meal to go **before** bringing it to the table. Simply raising your awareness at the table can go a long way toward preventing overeating. The following are some made-over meals from some popular restaurants. Mst are located in southern California but I think that they illustrate how to make over different types of meals if you keep the portion control in mind.

Burrito Mexicano with Chicken at Baja Fresh

Served: 3.5 ounces of chips, 300-calorie burrito

Madeover: 1 ounce of chips, 1/2 the burrito

I find it easier not to eat the chips because the actual act of eating them becomes unconscious. If you must, one ounce is about a handful.

Linguini a la Marinara with Grilled Chicken at Olive Garden

Served: 3 cups of pasta, 2 ounces of chicken, 2 breadsticks

Madeover: 1 cup pasta, 2 ounces of chicken, 1 breadstick

Vegetarian Pizza at Sbarro

Served: 10 ounces

Madeover: 5 ounces

By just cutting the slice in half and possibly sharing it with a friend, you will be less tempted to overeat.

Sample Week 15 Eating Out Goals:

I will create a game plan for my five favorite restaurants by looking up my favorite meals either on their menu or the Internet.

or

I will order within my preset game plan when I go out to eat.

or

I will only eat lunch and dinner out twice this week.

or

I will try to split my entrée with a friend or ask to have it split with half in a doggy bag.

Week 15 Your Eating Out Goals:

_____

_____

_____

_____

_____

_____

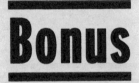

Bonus

Burn Calories

After you have been focusing on your eating habits for a long time, they will seem like old hat. You will lose weight and you will feel great. You started exercising but even that is feeling a bit stale. It doesn't help that you have hit your steady weight or setpoint. To push past this you need to increase the intensity of your exercise. You could coast through your cardio sessions. But to get a sleek, more lean-looking body, a leisurely stroll will only keep your physique at a standstill. The following are 16 workouts that will melt your body fat and have you turning heads in no time.

Inside the Gym

Treadmill. If you are suffering from treadmill boredom, you may want to use this workout from Chris McGrath, CSCS, CPT, in New York. "One of the reasons why I like to do this treadmill workout is pretty much everyone that I work with, even after they do it for 20 minutes or 30 minutes, is surprised how quickly the time went because most people find treadmills boring," says McGrath. "When it changes every single minute or two minutes, it gives you something to focus on as opposed to the same steady pace the whole time, plus it gives you a harder workout. Part of the purpose is to get you to an intensity that you couldn't maintain for more than a minute or two."

Start out walking at a reasonable pace using the incline, then each minute start bringing the incline up. McGrath starts out bringing it up a couple of levels. "Typically, I will start just flat then the next minute, I will bring it up to a 2.0 incline, next minute 4.0 and so on. And that usually gives them a gradual warm up for the first five minutes and gets their heart rate up," he says. Depending on your fitness level, continue increasing the incline while checking your heart rate. Continue doing that until you are at the higher end of your training zone. Once you get there and are working out at a higher intensity, usually in the first 10 minutes, continue to bring the heart rate up.

This is where McGrath gets creative with his client's workout. "I can gradually bring the heart rate back down. More often than not when someone is working out really hard at an incline of 12.0 or 15.0, I might bring them down to 6.0 so they have a recovery. Their heart rate comes down a little bit, their muscles get a little bit of a breather and work more normally for them again and then I will bring it up." So each minute, change the intensity. Bring it to a more moderate intensity so you can recover and then bring it up to a higher one — keep flopping it back and forth.

Rowing Machine. For a quick, 20-minute cardio session that will hit your whole body, use this suggestion from Dave Harris, CSCS, a strength and fitness con-

sultant in Toronto, Ontario, Canada. Warm
up for five minutes by biking or light jogging. Then jump on the ergometer or
rower, row for one minute as hard and as
fast as you possibly can. Then rest for two
minutes by rowing real easy and slow. Do
this six times.

Mix weights and cardio. Try this full-
body, boot camp workout designed by
Raymond Wallace, NASM-CPT, master
athletic trainer and coach at New York
Sports Club, to get you into fighting shape.

For the week you'll walk, run or bike
(preferably outdoors) for 45 minutes to an
hour, four times. Then you'll hit the gym
three times and do the strength-training
circuit on the next page. Do the exercises in
the order that they are listed. When needed, rest 30 to 90 seconds between sets. For
descriptions of how the exercises should be
done, they are available online at
www.muscle-fitness.com under the training link. Repeat each superset three times
before moving to the next one.

Exercise	Reps or Duration
Squat	15-20
with Jump Rope	1-2 minutes
Squat with	20
Overhead Press	
with Jump Rope	1-2 minutes
Alternating One-Arm	30-40
Bent-Over Rows	(15-20 reps each arm)
with "Double"	15-20 (each leg)
Walking Lunges	(don't alternate legs)
Alternating One-Arm	30-40
Lat Pulldowns	(15-20 reps each arm)
with Wall Squat Jumps	20
(jump and touch the highest point on a wall each time)	
Stability Ball Chest Presses	30
with Pushups	15
(pause 1 second at the bottom)	
Alternating Bicep Curls	30
(standing on one leg)	
with Dips off Bench	15
(feet resting on stability ball)	

Follow up with:

- 30 minutes of bike riding or step climbing training intervals
- Five to 10 minutes of ab training your choice
- Cooldown and stretch 10 minutes

Stationary bike. Spinning or indoor cycling class can give you a great interval cardio workout (and could do wonders for your social life if you attend enough). But if you're a class-phobic or you can't fit one into your schedule, you can simulate Ken Szekretar Jr.'s rides that he leads at the New York Sports Club: Keep the bike at a set resistance for five minutes. This is your flat section and you are going to build on your cadence (the amount of revolutions you are doing). Now pedal at a cadence that you will be able to maintain for a minute and then be able to incrementally increase two revolutions per minute for 20 minutes.

"Here's something you can do for resistance loading," says Szekretar. "I have [my class participants] start on the flat and then the hill gradually gets a slight grade. From there it gets a slight increase and then I will tell them to keep bringing that resistance heavier and heavier, sort of simulating an increased steepness in the hill."

Use three different cardio machines. You can turn a boring cardio workout into an indoor triathlon challenge using this "ironman" workout from Michelle Basta Boubion, NSCA-CPT and amateur triathlete. The total time of this workout is 40 minutes, although you can certainly increase the time by as much as 10 minutes, depending on your fitness level and your goals. "Make sure you recover sufficiently before starting the next interval," Boubion warns. "If necessary, instead of following the 1:1 work:rest ratio (that is outlined below), try a 1:1.5 work:rest ratio and repeat each cycle only three times. As you get stronger, decrease your rest time by a quarter, then half, of each work period."

Equipment	Workout Intensity	Time
Treadmill	Warm-up	5 minutes
Treadmill	Medium	1 minute
	High	1 minute

Continue to alternate between work and recovery in one-minute segments for four more cycles, for a total of 10 minutes.

Elliptical Trainer	Medium	1 minute
	High	1 minute

Continue to alternate between work and recovery in one-minute segments for four more cycles, for a total of 10 minutes.

Stationary Bike	Medium	1 minute
	High	1 minute

Continue to alternate between work and recovery in one minute-segments for four more cycles, for a total of 10 minutes.

Stationary Bike	Cool Down	5 minutes

Outside or At-Home Workouts

Take to the Track. Wind sprints may sound like a breeze but this high-intensity activity will raise your heart rate and make your body use those fat stores in a minimal amount of time.

Try the following drill from Harris: Warm up for five minutes by biking or light jogging. "It is important to make sure that your Achilles tendon and hamstrings are properly warmed up to avoid injury," says Harris. Sprint for 50 seconds or about 300 meters. Then walk back to your starting place. This active rest period should last no longer than 120 seconds. Repeat six times.

Bicycle Race. It's a race against yourself today as you take to the streets or bike trails of your town. After a leisurely 10-minute ride, pick a starting point that you'll remember. Now choose a time in your head: 20 minutes if you're a relative beginner, up to 30 or more if you're an expert rider. You're going to ride for that amount of time through any course you wish, although you should make sure that the terrain, if not flat, has as many "ups" as "downs." See how far you can get in your chosen time, stop and rest two to five minutes, then turn around, reset the clock and retrace your route. Your goal? To go farther in the same amount of time by passing your original starting point. Once you finish, take 10 minutes to return to your original starting place at a slower cool-down pace.

Take the stairs. Use this trio of approaches to make this challenging activity a bit more work. First, walk or run up the stairs one step at a time, then walk down. Second, walk or run up the stairs two steps at a time (hitting every other one). Again walk down, using the time as your recovery period. Third, do stair stakes, jumping side to side from one step to the next. To do this you will jump to your right, landing on your right foot, left foot slightly behind you. Then jump to your left and onto the next step, landing on your left foot. Again, walk down. Continue repeating the sequence for 30 minutes.

Athletic Drills. Remember high school PE class? Whether you liked it or not, it did offer up options to the fat-burning boredom. Try these drills to get your heart pumping and maybe you will discover the love of the game again.

• **High Knees/Squat Thrusts:** Run in place as fast as you can with your knees high to your waist for two minutes. Stop, squat to the ground with your hands by your feet and thrust your legs out behind you so you're in a push-up position. Return to the squat position and then stand. Do this 15 times. Repeat the cycle of running, squatting and thrusting five times.

• **Soccer Dribbling:** Kick a soccer ball

back and forth from foot to foot while walking, then jogging. Move up and down a field. If possible, run forward in an S-pattern with the ball. Complete 10 up-and-back laps of a soccer field or large grassy area.

• **Line Sprints:** Find a tennis or basketball court or make your own lines in a field (six lines spaced 6 yards apart). Start at the first line and run to the next nearest line. Bend down and touch it, then run back to your starting mark. Touch that line, sprint to the second line, touch it and sprint back to the start. Repeat this process until you've touched all the lines. Take a one-minute rest after completing each full set of sprints. For your second set, run to the first line, stop and then run backward to the starting point. Repeat this sequence for all lines. Repeat the line drills for 20 minutes.

Take to the hills! This workout is inspired by the one Andre Agassi used to jack up his fitness levels. For this, you'll simply need a relatively steep hill, a stopwatch and some sturdy shoes with traction. Start with a five-minute light jog on flat terrain, then it's time to work: From a point at the bottom of the hill, hit the stopwatch and sprint full-force straight to the top. Stop the watch and note your time, then either walk briskly or, if you're more of an advanced athlete (and don't suffer from knee problems), jog lightly to the bottom. Continue with four to nine more sprints, depending on your fitness levels, and keep note of your best time, which you should try to beat next time you do the workout. Finish with a slow jog on a flat surface for five minutes to cool down.

Three things at once? The typical triathlon is a swim, bike ride and run, but who says that lineup is a hard-and-fast rule? Make up your own triathlon this weekend, based on your favorite activities. Rollerblade, bike and shoot hoops. Or perhaps run stairs, jump rope and swim. You can pick either a time period or a distance for each activity.

Park-Bench Obstacle Course. Head to the park for a running and resistance-training combo designed to work your muscles and burn some serious calories. If the park doesn't have benches spaced at least 12 yards apart, you can also use the bench of a picnic table or any low, sturdy object. After a five-minute light jog, start at the first bench with 30 seconds of step-ups. Then run to the next bench and perform 30 seconds of push-ups. Go to a third bench and do 30 seconds of squats, then run to a fourth bench and perform triceps dips for, you guessed it, 30 seconds. Rest 30 to 60 seconds and repeat. Complete the circuit 10 times total and finish with a light five-minute jog.

• **Step-Up:** Start with your feet together in front of the bench; step up with your right leg onto the bench and lift your body to bring your left leg to meet your right. Return to the ground and repeat with your left leg.

• **Push-Up:** Place your hands outside shoulder-width on the bench, keep your legs straight out behind you and lower yourself from an arms-straight position to an elbows-bent position.

• **Squat:** Stand upright, place your hands on your hips or shoulders and bend your knees while shifting your hips back until your butt lightly touches the seat of the bench. Return to a standing position and repeat.

• **Triceps Dip:** Sit on the bench with your hands next to your hips, knuckles facing out. Walk your feet out, bring your butt off the bench and start dipping, bending your elbows until your upper arms are parallel with the ground then returning to the arms-extended position for reps.

Almost Anywhere

Skip 'N' Kick. Kick, skip and shuffle your way to a cardio workout on Tuesday, courtesy of a quick program by Chris McGrath, CSCS, CPT, a master trainer with New York Sports Club. "It's designed to get you moving in every different direction and get your heart rate up," he says. Start by marking off a 20-yard line in a field or the backyard (you can also use a marked football field). Start at one end and go 20 yards doing butt kicks, stop for five seconds, then return to the start, again doing butt kicks. Repeat the drill with high-knee raises next, power skips for the third go-round and finish with side shuffles. Repeat the four-pronged drill 20 times. If you're more advanced go for more drills, or extend the yardage for each drill.

• **Butt Kick:** Run with an exaggerated leg kick, coming close or touching your glutes with your foot.

• **High-Knee Raise:** Run while exaggerating your knee lift.

• **Power Skip:** Skip with a strong forward motion with both your arms and legs.

• **Side Shuffle:** Turn sideways and bring your feet together and apart to move laterally.

Jump rope. For only a few bucks, you can buy an inexpensive jump rope and throw it in your gym bag, briefcase or suitcase. Jumping rope is a major calorie burner, too. Use this high-powered workout from Bobby Aldridge, LWMC, CPT, fitness consultant and owner/operator of Senergy Fitness Systems, a personal training company based in Atlanta. Jump for three to five minutes and rest for 30 to 60 seconds. Do this for a total of 20to 30 minutes. "Since this is an interval-type program, 30 minutes is probably long enough to get an incredible workout," Aldridge says. "If you want to make this routine even more challenging, instead of resting, hold your rope in one hand and do small jumps in place for the allotted 'rest' time."

Step to it! These drills will develop power, strength and agility while burning fat fast.

Stand with a box, or a step, that is at least a foot tall, in front of you. Step up and down on the box for five minutes to warm up. Then, standing with the box in front of you, jump up on top of the box bringing your knees up to your chest. Then jump back down to the start. Repeat 10 times. Rest for 30 seconds then move to the right of the bench, jumping on top of the box as before. Repeat 10 times. Rest for 30 seconds then move to the left of the bench and do the same, also 10 times. After resting for 60 seconds, repeat the front, right, left cycle for 20 minutes.

For more of a unilateral approach, use McGrath's variation: Stand to the left of a step on your left leg, then jump on to the top of the box landing on your right leg. Repeat for 15 seconds. Rest for 10 seconds, then change sides and legs. Continue this cycle until fatigued. To make this variation more challenging, make your landing leg the same as your jumping leg.

To push the anaerobic threshold (to build cardiovascular health) on any of the drills above, McGrath suggests varying the explosiveness of your jumps. For example, do five seconds of less explosive jumping, then do 15 seconds of more explosive jumping, alternating back and forth until you are fatigued.

10,000 Steps. You'll want to visit a sports store and pick up a pedometer for this one. Don't worry, they're inexpensive (as little as $10-$40) and you may find it's one of the best investments you've ever made for your health. On Thursday, from the time you get up to the time you go to bed, you'll don the pedometer and aim to take at least 10,000 steps throughout the day. Go out of your way to get steps — choose the stairs over the elevator, park the car farther away in the lot if you go to the store, take a walk during lunch or after work. The pedometer gives you a concrete goal to pursue and you'll find yourself actively seeking ways to get extra steps. Careful: This particular workout may be addictive!

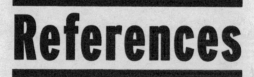

References

Alagoz, M.S., Basterzi, A.D., Uysal, A.C., Tuzer, V., et al. The psychiatric view of patients of aesthetic surgery: Self-esteem, body image and eating attitude. *Aesthetic Plastic Surgery* 27: 345-348, 2003.

Allen, JE. Dieting's ups and downs: the frequent gaining and shedding of pounds may weaken the body's immune system. For girls, physical development could be affected. *Los Angeles Times*. Internet. Available 21 June 2004. http://www.latimes.com/features/health/la-he-yoyo21jun21.1.245050.story?coll=la-headlines-health

Almiron-Roig E, Drewnowski A. Hunger, thirst and energy intakes following consumption of caloric beverages. *Physiology & Behavior* 79: 767-773, 2003.

Anderson, GH, Woodend, D. Consumption of sugars and the regulation of short-term satiety and food intake. *Am J Clin Nutr* 78: 843S-849S, 2003.

Blair SN, LaMonte MJ, Nichaman MZ. The evolution of physical activity recommendations: how much is enough? *Am J Clin Nutr* 79: 913S-920S, 2004.

Bogers RP, Brug J, van Assema P, Dagnelie PC. Explaining fruit and vegetable consumption: the theory of planned behavior and misconception of personal intake levels. *Appetite* 42: 157-166, 2004.

Bowman SA, Vinyard BT. Fast food consumption of US adults: Impact on energy and nutrient intakes and overweight status. *J Am Col Nutr* 23: 163-168, 2004.

Buchowski MS, Acra S, Majchrzak KM, Sun M, Chen KY. Patterns of physical activity in free-living adults in the southern United States. *Eur J Clin Nutr* 58: 828-837, 2004.

Clifton PM, Noakes M, Sullivan D, Erichsen N, Ross D, Annison, Fassoulakis A, Cehun M, Nestel

P. Cholesterol-lowering effects of plant sterol esters differ in milk, bread and cereal. *Eur J Clin Nutr* 58: 503-509, 2004.

Davis C, Strachan S, Berkson M. Sensitivity to reward: implications for overeating and overweight. *Appetite* 42: 131-138, 2004.

Davis, JL. Yo-yo dieting may hurt immunity: weight loss via crash diets many increase infections. *WebMD Medical News.* June 3, 2004.

Devitt AA, Mattes RD. Effects of food unit size and energy density on intake in humans. *Appetite* 42: 213-220, 2004.

Diliberti, N, Bordi, PL, Conklin, MT, Roe, LS, Rolls, BJ. Increases portion size leads to increases energy intake in a restaurant meal. *Obesity Research* 12: 562-568, 2004.

Elliot T. Water guidelines are all wet. *Muscle & Fitness,* June 2004.

Field AE, Manson JE, Laird N, Williamson DF, Willett WC, Colditz GA. Weight cycling and the risk of developing type 2 diabetes among adult women in the United States. *Obesity Research* 12: 267-274, 2004.

Hannum SM, Carson LA, Evans EM, Canene KA, Petr EL, Bui L, Erdman JW. Use of portion-controlled entrees enhances weight loss in women. *Obesity Research* 12: 538-546, 2004.

Hill, A.J., Franklin, J.A., Mothers, daughters and dieting: investigating the transmission of weight control. *British Journal of Clinical Psychology* 37:3-13, 1998.

Hill, A.J., Pallin, V. Dieting awareness and low self-worth: related issues in 8-year-old girls. *International Journal of Eating Disorders* 24: 405-413, 1998.

Hoolihan, L. Beyond Calcium: The protective

attributes of dairy products and their constituents. *Nutrition Today* 39: 69-75, 2004.

Janssen I, Katzmarzyk PT, Ross R, Leon AS, Skinner JS, Rao DC, Wilmore JH, Raninen T, Bouchard C. Fitness alters the associations of BMI and waist circumference with total abdominal fat. *Obesity Research* 12: 525-537, 2004.

Jeffrey RW, Wing RR, Sherwood NE, Tate DF. Physical activity and weight loss: does prescribing higher physical activity goals improve outcome? *Am J Clin Nutr* 78: 684-689, 2003.

Jenkins, DJA, Kendal, CWC, Marchie, A, Augustin, LSA. Too much sugar, too much carbohydrate, or just too much? *Am J Clin Nutr* 78: 843S-849S, 2003.

Juntunen KS, Laaksonen DE, Autio K, Niskanen LK, Holst JJ, Savolainen KE, Liukkonen K-H, Poutanen KS, Mykkanen HM. Structural differences between rye and wheat breads but not total fiber content may explain the lower postprandial insulin response to rye bread. *Am J Clin Nutr* 78: 957-964, 2003.

Koh-Banerjee P, Chu N-F, Spiegelman D, Rosner B, Colditz G, Willett W, Rimm E. Prospective study of the association of changes in dietary intake, physical activity, alcohol consumption and smoking with 9-y gain in waist circumference among 16,587 U.S. men. *Am J Clin Nutr* 78: 719-727, 2003.

Kiefer I, Prock P, Lawrence C, Eng B, Wise J, Bieger W, Bayer P, Psych M, Rathmanner T, Kunze M, Rieder A. Supplementation with mixed fruit and vegetable juice concentrates increased serum antioxidants and folate in healthy adults. *J Am Col Nutr* 23: 205-211, 2004.

Kral TVE, Roe LS, Rolls BJ. Combined effects of energy density and portion size on energy intake in women. *Am J Clin Nutr* 79: 962-968, 2004.

Krumm, JE. The Sweetest Taboo: Are you desperately seeking sugar? Here's how you can have your cake –and stay on your diet too. *Muscle & Fitness Hers*, 38-42, April 2003.

Kluger, J. Why We Eat. For social reasons: For humans, food does more than merely nourish. It socializes — and civilizes — us as well. *TIME*. June 7, 2004, 72.

Lackey CJ, Kolasa KM. Healthy Eating: Defining the nutrient quality of foods. *Nutrition Today* 39:26-29, 2004.

Laliberte R. Distilling the water myth. *Shape* May: 136-140, 2004.

Landers P, Wolfe MM, Glore S, Guild R, Phillips L. Effect of weight loss plans on body composition and diet duration. Abstract. J Okla State Med Assoc. 95: 329-331, 2002.

Levine AS, Kotz CM, Gosnell. Sugars: hedonic aspects, neuroregulation and energy balance. *Am J Clin Nutr* 78: 834S-842S, 2003.

Miller Jones J, Reicks M, Adams J, Fulcher G, Marguart L. Becoming proactive with the whole-grain message. *Nutrition Today* 39: 10-16, 2004.

Murphy, SP, Johnston, RK. The science basis of recent US guidance on sugars intake. *Am J Clin Nutr* 79: 711-712, 2004.

Nicklas, TA, O'Neil, C, Myers L. the Importance of breakfast consumption to nutrition of children, adolescents and young adults. *Nutrition Today* 39: 30-38, 2004.

Nocton, A-M. Dairy and Your Diet. *Muscle & Fitness Hers* 4:74-78, 2003.

Pliner P, Mann N. Influence of social norms and palatability on amount consumed and food choice. *Appetite* 42: 227-237, 2004.

Popkin, BM, Nielsen, SJ. The Sweetening of the World's Diet. *Obesity Research* 11: 1325-1332, 2003.

Prince JR. Why all the fuss about portion size? Designing the "New American Plate." *Nutrition Today* 39: 59-63, 2004.

Roan S. Calcium connection: Foods rich in the nutrient might help people shed pounds, but more research is needed. *Los Angeles Times*. Online. Internet. Available 21 June 2004. http://www.latimes.com/features/health/la-he-calcium21jun21.story

Saris, WHM. Sugars, energy metabolism and body weight control. *Am J Clin Nutr* 78: 850S-857S, 2003.

Schenk S, Davidson CJ, Zderic TW, Byerley LO, Coyle EF. Different glycemic indexes of breakfast cereals are not due to glucose entry into blood but to glucose removal by tissue. *Am J Clin Nutr* 78: 742-748, 2003.

Schoeller DA. But how much physical activity? *Am J Clin Nutr* 78: 669-670, 2003.

Schwartz, D.J., Phares, V., Tantleff-Dunn, S., Thompson, J.K. Body image, psychological functioning and parental feedback regarding physical appearance. *International Journal of Eating Disorders* 25: 339-343, 1999.

Sigman-Grant, M, Morita, J. Defining and interpreting intakes of sugars. *Am J Clin Nutr* 78: 815S-826S, 2003.

Smith AT, Kuznesof S, Richardson DP, Seal CJ. Behavioural, attitudinal and dietary responses to the consumption of wholegrain foods. *Proc Nutr Soc* 62: 455-467, 2003.

Smolak, L., Levine, M.P., Schremer, F. Parental input and weight concerns among elementary school children. *International Journal of Eating Disorders* 25: 263-271, 1999.

Sonnenburg B, Barke S. Size does matter. *Muscle & Fitness Hers* 64-71, April 2003.

Thompson, J.K., Heinberg, L.J., Altabe, M., and Tantleff-Dunn, S. Exacting Beauty:Theory, Assessment, and Treatment of Body Image Disturbance. American Psychological Association: Washington, D.C. 1999, p. 202-204.

Tucker KL, Olson B, Bakun P, Dallal GE, Selhub J, Rosenberg IH. Breakfast cereal fortified with folic acid, vitamin B-6 and vitamin B-12 increases vitamin concentrations and reduces homocysteine concentrations: a randomized trial. *Am J Clin Nutr* 79: 805-811, 2004.

Wein, D. Rise and Shine. *Muscle & Fitness Hers,* 44-47, October/ November 2001.

Zemel MB. Role of calcium and dairy products in energy partitioning and weight management. *Am J Clin Nutr* 79: 907S-912S, 2004.

Zemel MB, Thompson W, Milstead A, Morris K, Campbell P. Calcium and dairy acceleration of weight and fat loss during energy restriction in obese adults. *Obesity Research* 12: 582-590, 2004.

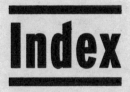

NO MORE DIETS ... EVER

Order These Great True Crime Books:

Please send the books checked below:

	Price Ea.	Qty.	Total
☐ *Sex, Power & Murder* — Chandra Levy and Gary Condit: the affair that shocked America	$5.99		
☐ *They're Killing Our Children* — Inside the kidnapping and child murder epidemic sweeping America	$6.99		
☐ *JonBenet* — The police files	$7.99		
☐ *Sixteen Minutes From Home* — The Columbia Space Shuttle tragedy	$5.99		
☐ *Saddam* — The face of evil	$5.99		
☐ *The Murder of Laci Peterson*	$5.99		
☐ *Diana* — Secrets & Lies	$5.99		
☐ *Martha Stewart* — Just Desserts	$6.99		
☐ *Driven to Kill* — The Clara Harris story	$5.99		

Postage & Handling:
U.S., $ 2.75 for one book, $ 1.00 for each additional

Total enclosed:

Ship to:

NAME _____

ADDRESS _____

CITY _____ STATE _____ ZIP _____

Please make your check or money order payable to AMI Books and mail it along with this order form to AMI Mail Order Books, 1000 American Media Way, Boca Raton, FL 33464-1000. Allow 4-6 weeks for delivery. Payable in U.S. funds only. No cash or COD accepted. We accept check or money orders ($15.00 fee for returned check). **Offer not available in Canada.**

0904NMDE

Order These Great Celebrity Books:

Please send the books checked below:

Order These Great
Health & Fitness Books:

Please send the books checked below:

	Price Ea.	Qty.	Total
☐ *Instant Weight Loss* — Lose 10 pounds in 10 days — and keep it off!	$5.99		
Postage & Handling: U.S., $ 2.75 for one book, $ 1.00 for each additional			
Total enclosed:			

Ship to:

NAME _____

ADDRESS _____

CITY _____ STATE _____ ZIP _____